Vera Miguelote

# Doctors, medicines and the market

Vera Miguelote

# Doctors, medicines and the market

## The power of the pharmaceutical industry?

ScienciaScripts

**Imprint**



Cover image: www.ingimage.com

This book is a translation from the original published under ISBN 978-3-330-75344-0.

Publisher:
Sciencia Scripts
is a trademark of
Dodo Books Indian Ocean Ltd. and OmniScriptum S.R.L publishing group

120 High Road, East Finchley, London, N2 9ED, United Kingdom
Str. Armeneasca 28/1, office 1, Chisinau MD-2012, Republic of Moldova, Europe
Printed at: see last page
**ISBN: 978-620-8-04600-2**

*To my daughters Flavia, Carla and Claudia,*
*for the importance of their existence in my life*

## Thanks

This book is the result of my master's thesis at the Institute of Social Medicine (IMS) of the State University of Rio de Janeiro (UERJ) and would not have been possible without some precious contributions. In this sense, I would like to thank Professor Kenneth Camargo, my advisor, for his academic support, consistent discourse and affectionate mastery along the way. I would also like to thank the other professors at IMS, especially Anna Maria Campos, Jane Sayd, Rosangela Caetano, George Kornis and Rubem Mattos, for their important academic contributions. I would also like to thank my dear daughter Carla, for her careful proofreading of the text, and my dear nephew Vinicius Guimaraes, graphic designer, for his precious aesthetic interventions. And finally, to the doctors interviewed, for their willingness to collaborate with the research and for sharing their experiences.

*The role of the intellectual is no longer [...] to tell everyone's mute truth; rather, it is to fight against the forms of power precisely where he is both the object and the instrument: in the order of knowledge, "truth", "consciousness" and discourse.*

*Michel Foucault.*

# Index


| | |
|---|---|
| Chapter 1 | 12 |
| Chapter 2 | 17 |
| Chapter 3 | 29 |
| Chapter 4 | 38 |
| Chapter 5 | 51 |

# Preface

## Health, knowledge and the market, the conflictive coexistence

One of the most significant changes in the historical development of the scientific field was the emergence of the so-called *"Big Science"*. Experimental science ceased to be within the reach of individual researchers and progressively became a large-scale enterprise, requiring major investments and a long maturation period.

This phenomenon is reflected in the relationship between science and technology, particularly in the relatively recent dominance of contemporary pharmaceuticals, which began practically at the same time as the 20th century and also became *"Big Business"* after the Second World War.

The commercial nature of the pharmaceutical enterprise inevitably creates friction with the normative ideals, at least as formally expressed in its deontology, which guide the field of health interventions. If "health" is a right, it is neither ethical nor moral for economic barriers to prevent or distort access to goods and services of this kind for those who need them.

State regulation is, in general, the resource that allows citizens to curb distortions and guarantee equal access to such goods and services, which inevitably leads to such regulation being seen as an obstacle to the full realization of the lucrative potential of investment in research and development in health-related sectors.

We have a double dilemma here: on the one hand, the possibility of imposing high prices, restricting the benefits of certain health interventions to a select few; on the other hand, the pressure to overuse other interventions as a way of guaranteeing the profitability of the investment made.

These two basic aspects are multiplied in a variety of strategies, such as the use of patent legislation to extend monopolies indefinitely; the masking of advertising costs as "research"; undue or misleading advertising; the enticement, explicit or not, of health professionals, "opinion leaders", as marketing spearheads, among many others. Authors such as Marcia Angell and Ben Goldacre have documented, in publications accessible to the general public, the use of such strategies by the pharmaceutical industry to guarantee its profits and market growth. This process, however, is not without its problems. There is a permanent tension in health agencies, especially in the medical sphere, between the need to maintain the legitimacy of doctors and medicines, and to maximize profits.

There is, however, a specific aspect of these strategies in relation to the pharmaceutical industry, which is the articulation of research and the dissemination of knowledge with the commercial interests already mentioned. The pharmaceutical industry needs to sell drugs, the publishing industry needs to sell magazine subscriptions and/or advertising space, and knowledge about the use of medication articulates these interests. The whole cycle of production and dissemination of knowledge in this area is controlled by and subject to commercial interests, which in turn, as we have seen, are not necessarily aligned with the interests and needs of the general population. The latter, in turn, although without necessarily having a clear view of this dynamic, view the alliances established within the medical industrial complex with suspicion.

With the growing use of internet-mediated communication, especially the so-called "internet 2.0" and its "social networks", it is not difficult to find examples of criticism, although sometimes little more than conspiracy theories, of the perceived predominance of economic interest over any other value. It is claimed, for example, that "the cure for cancer" is only not available because it is hidden by the pharmaceutical industry, which would "lose market share" if such a panacea were released to everyone. It doesn't matter here how absurd this conspiracy theory is; the mere fact that you can find someone willing to believe in it shows what was said at the end of the previous paragraph.

And herein lies a problem. Despite the inevitable distortions, medicines are an indispensable input for health care. They are effective tools in relieving and even eliminating some suffering; the introduction of antibiotics was a real revolution in the treatment of infectious diseases, saving countless lives, and the same can recently be said of antiretrovirals. Health *experts* are forced to use, and defend, a product from an industrial sector that demonstrably engages in improper practices when promoting its sales. The logic of making the most profit in the shortest time casts a shadow of suspicion over the industry and the medical *establishment* that compromises the necessary credibility with the population, with damaging consequences for everyone.

The answer to this dilemma is to have more, not less, science, more critical eyes looking at the field of biomedical knowledge production, as a way of guaranteeing its integrity. This principle is behind initiatives such as the UK's AllTrials, led by the aforementioned Ben Goldacre, which proposes that all the raw data from all clinical trials be made freely available, so that they can be analyzed by independent researchers, guaranteeing the quality and reliability of the results.

Vera's work is therefore both a denunciation and a proposal, making clear the need for research and professional training in health, and particularly in medicine, to be independent from the commercial interests of the biomedical knowledge industry. This depends not only on the quality of and access to the work of these professionals, but also on their legitimacy vis-à-vis society in general.

It is in this sense that we have been working over the last few years to produce critical studies on knowledge in the Social Studies Group on Health Technoscience/BioMedSci at the Institute of Social Medicine at UERJ, to expose the cogs of the knowledge industry as a contribution to its improvement and subordinate to the ethical and political values that underlie any therapeutic project. Vera Miguelote's work, which I had the pleasure and honor of supervising, is part of this matrix. Vera leads us through deep theoretical reflection in the company of key authors such as Foucault and Fleck, to a better understanding of the complex dynamics of knowledge production and its interaction with industrial production, showing the often implicit determinants that underlie such dynamics. In particular, its empirical investigation with doctors/teachers at a university hospital exposes the pitfalls posed by the insertion of pharmaceutical industry interests in this environment. The great fragility of the professional in the face of the power and enticement of industrial giants is evident, calling into question the narratives that establish the professional category of doctors as the "imperial power" of health, corroborating the findings of Peter Conrad in his research on medicalization. Carrying out "research" that is actually just another marketing strategy ties professional development and prestige to this strategy.

Rio de Janeiro, February 15, 2017

Kenneth Rochel de Camargo Jr., MD PhD

Associate Professor - Senior Associate Professor Instituto de Medicina Social - Social Medicine Institute Universidade do Estado do Rio de Janeiro - Rio de Janeiro State U. (Brazil) Editor - Physis http://www.scielo.br/physisAssociate Editor - American Journal of Public Health e-mail: kenneth@uerj.br

# Introduction

This work is part of my interest, as a psychiatrist, in understanding the medical condition in today's world. Related to the foundations of medicine and its implications for clinical practice, this interest resulted from discussions of the theoretical content of some of the courses I took during my master's degree in Collective Health at the Institute of Social Medicine of the State University of Rio de Janeiro (UERJ), especially the courses aimed at studying the construction of medical knowledge. When I realized that an important part of research activities is under the control of the commercial interests of the pharmaceutical industry, I understood that the collaboration of doctors in the industry's research projects implied a co-production of knowledge. The aim of this book is therefore to help us understand the role played by doctors in their relationship with the industry.

The relevance of the topic and the logic of the approach are outlined in the first chapter, through a selective literature review on the subject. The second, third and fourth chapters are my pillars of theoretical support.

The second, entitled "The medical knowledge industry: A powerful cog in the wheel", looks at the context of a macro-political cog in which the pharmaceutical industry is linked to the "industry" of knowledge, conditioning the construction and dissemination of biomedical knowledge to the same logic as the capitalist production and distribution of merchandise. Configuring a powerful direction for economic interests, a set of strategic techniques guarantees the consumption of medicines at the same time as encouraging the production and dissemination of scientific articles. Used to lend credibility to results of interest to them, the pharmaceutical industry's investment in research funding has transformed the process of scientific legitimization into a marketing strategy.

The third chapter, "Power-knowledge: an inseparable link", analyzes contemporary power relations with the aim of understanding the micropolitical dimension of the medical knowledge production process. It is based on Foucault's (1995) conception of power in order to understand, in the biopolitical dimension of society, the force of the economic power of industry - which, strategically using the articulation of knowledge/power, is dominant in the contemporary configuration.

In the fourth chapter, the epistemological dimension of the knowledge-power relationship is based on Fleck's (1979) concepts - *thought collective* and *thought style* - in order to attribute contemporary medical discourse to facilitating the pharmaceutical industry's marketing strategies. From a contemporary biopolitical perspective, the pharmaceutical industry's investment in clinical research projects is the result of a reconfiguration of forces. In this sense, the articulation of epistemological aspects with economic interests should be understood as a strategic position of power.

The fifth chapter deals with a field study carried out in a university hospital. It presents the study methodology and the analysis and discussion of the results. Of a qualitative nature, the method of semi-structured interviews was used as a tool for investigating the interaction between doctors and the research funding industry. Information was collected from four doctors, professors of medicine, who were co-participants in research projects funded by the pharmaceutical industry. In the thematic evaluation, three recurring themes were selected: the way in which doctors are involved in research, the process of constructing clinical evidence and doctors' understanding of the contemporary construction of knowledge.

The analysis and discussion of the results are based on the themes listed above. Through the empirical analysis of this material, two perspectives of evaluation are developed: the first relates to the way in which the pharmaceutical industry, as financier, coordinates and directs research, and the second refers to the way in which prescribing doctors are understanding the contemporary production of medical knowledge.

Finally, conclusions are drawn about the interaction between medical research collaborators and the funding industry in the processes of co-production of medical knowledge.

## 1 Linking Scientific Knowledge and Industry Pharmaceuticals: A Historical Overview

As a result of the major economic changes and huge technological advances that have taken place in recent decades, the technical-scientific medical discourse has become linked to economic development, transforming medicine into a territory dominated by capitalist and mercantilist forms.

Science began to link up with industry when the first chemotherapy drug was developed from research into a dye tolerated by the human body (late 19th and early 20th centuries). Pharmacology was developed by Paul Ehrlich; in 1904, with Trypan's red, against trypanosomes and, in 1910, with Salvarsan, an arsenical compound effective against syphilis. At this point, scientifically-based therapeutics emerged, which was definitively consolidated with the synthesis of the first sulfa drugs in 1937. Thus, the birth of fine chemistry marked the beginning of the development of the pharmaceutical industry (SAYD, 1998).

With the advent of war, scientific knowledge advanced: on the one hand, science discovered antibiotics, indispensable for the survival of soldiers; on the other hand, technology changed the history of armed conflict by creating ever more powerful and effective weapons for its gruesome task. History therefore reveals a scientific production that was closely linked to the military, against the backdrop of industrial production (BERNAL, 1964).

Hochman's (2002) study on the relationship between the scientific world and capitalist dynamics overcame theoretical and methodological differences between various authors (Khun, Bourdieu, Latour and Knorr-Cetina) and managed to integrate the concepts of scientific community, market, credibility and transepistemic arena. Considering this integration, the production of knowledge is configured as a special case of capitalist commodity production and distribution. With this assumption, science can only be understood from the social determination of its content

(BOURDIEU, 2005).

Despite the multiplicity of interests in the scientific world, credibility in science is conferred in the field of research: the main forum for validating knowledge. To the extent that economic production has come to depend on this value, legitimizing knowledge through research has gained prominence in political and economic negotiations. Knowledge, clothed in scientificity, became one of the pharmaceutical industry's main marketing strategies. It was in this context that the industry emerged as a funder of research and seized the possibility of directing interests in the biomedical area.

However, according to Angell (2007, p. 37), although bringing a drug to market is hard and time-consuming work, the pharmaceutical industries "do not nearly play the role in research and development (R&D) that they would like the public to believe". The pharmaceutical industry's participation in basic research, for example, amounts to an eighth of the total funding. Predominantly funded by the public service, the production of this type of research is "almost always carried out in universities or government research laboratories, either in the US or abroad" (ANGELL, 2007, p. 38).

The fundamental discoveries take place in basic research; researchers identify at the cellular level at which point in the physio-pathological chain the disease can be combated by a pharmacological agent. Although this is the longest and most difficult part of R&D, the large pharmaceutical industries contribute very little. The development phase is divided into two stages: pre-clinical and clinical. Pre-clinical research corresponds to the process of synthesizing and developing a substance, in order to verify that the molecules being studied have the properties identified in the basic research. This is where the pharmaceutical industry starts to get involved (ANGELL, 2007).

The industry keeps huge archives of drug candidate molecules. In pre-clinical development, after identification by computerized methods, the molecules are synthesized or extracted from animal, plant or mineral sources. Only a small proportion of drug candidate molecules make it through development and on to the all-important stage of clinical trials on human beings. Through successive clinical and epidemiological evaluations, the product is tested on a larger and larger scale to verify efficacy, cost/benefit aspects and side effects. Subjected to scientific and credible criteria, it is this research that legitimizes the product to obtain a license for the treatment of specific diseases.

The effective area of activity for the pharmaceutical industry is the clinical trials stage, i.e. the cutting edge of development. Paradoxically, although it is the least creative part of the process, clinical trials are the most expensive. The approval of a drug requires three phases of the clinical trials stage:

Phase I: with a small number of volunteers categorized as normal.

Phase II: involves hundreds of patients with the relevant disease or medical condition, whose outcome is compared with a similar group of patients not receiving the drug.

Phase III: evaluates the safety and efficacy of the drug in thousands of patients (ANGELL, 2007, p. 43).

Although the majority of industry-sponsored clinical trials are to test new drugs or procedures, many of them are of drugs already on sale - called "post-marketing" or "Phase IV" studies. In order to expand the market, these studies are looking for new uses for old drugs.

There are already studies that point to the possibility of a biased nature in these clinical trials funded by the pharmaceutical industry. The "need" to scientifically legitimize results of economic interest has led to the possibility of investing in the production of knowledge, but also in the selective publication of results (ANGELL, 2007). Configuring the knowledge industry, this mechanism will be discussed in the second chapter. It is a dynamic through which a large part of research activities, as well as the production and distribution of biomedical knowledge, is under the control of private commercial interests.

Given the importance of knowledge in the decision-making process, doctors keep up to date with research reports that feed into the medical literature. Bearing in mind that scientific production is increasingly subjugated to the interests of industry, this context points to distortions involving conflicts of interest and abuses of power.

Recent literature has highlighted the pharmaceutical industry's interest in promoting its products through its interaction with medical education and research. Although not typically promotional activities, medical refresher courses, continuing education and programs aimed at residents have often been funded by the pharmaceutical industry. To the extent that academic representation lends credibility to these activities, the participation of university professors has become part of the industry's marketing strategies (STEINMAN, BERO, CHREN, LANDERFELD, 2006).

In general, the latest recommendations, presented as advances in medical care, are disseminated by speakers funded by the pharmaceutical industry, presented as *experts,* with significant credentials in prestigious academic medical centers. Considering that, for the majority of doctors, participation in continuing education programs has become mandatory, and the pharmaceutical industries have begun to act to persuade doctors to change their prescribing practices, Abramson (2005) highlights his concern about this process.

The pharmaceutical industry invests specifically in medical staff. With enormous economic power, it offers a wide variety of incentives: promotion of events, travel expenses, hotels, gifts, books and advertising pamphlets, etc. Companies monitor doctors' preferences, habits and desires. A professor of Clinical Medicine at the Federal University of Sao Paulo reports, in an article in Epoca magazine (Nov. 2007), that when the advertiser found out he was a Corinthian, he offered tickets to an important match, with the right to a tribune of honor and food and drink. Because of cases like this, the issue of conflict of interest has been the subject of articles in magazines and journals.

Funded by the European Commission, the *lobby* group *Consumers International* published a study in London in October 2007 called *"Drugs, doctors and dinners: How drug companies influence health in the developing world",* pointing out the ethical failings of Europe's main pharmaceutical industries. After noting that, between 1995 and 2005, investment in marketing was double that in research, the study denounces the strategic marketing tactics aimed at doctors. The report considers that the doctor's opinion of a given pharmaceutical product not only influences but also determines its sales success. As a result, in developing countries, doctors have become the main target of pharmaceutical companies' promotional activities.

A study coordinated by researcher Eric Campbell, published in *The New England Journal of Medicine* (Oct/2007), on the influence of the industry on medical practice, concludes that although many professionals deny that receiving gifts influences prescriptions, 94% of doctors have some kind of relationship with the pharmaceutical industry (Revista Epoca, Nov/2007, p. 114).

It is in this context of conflicting interests that the interaction between the pharmaceutical industry and the research collaborator takes place, involving ethical, political and scientific issues. This research is based on the aspects listed above in order to: investigate how the doctor is included in the research process funded by the pharmaceutical industry; analyze the dynamics of the clinical evidence building processes developed by this industry; and evaluate the dissemination and assimilation of medical knowledge produced from these research processes.

## 2 The Medical Knowledge Industry: A Powerful Gear

There is a powerful mechanism through which the pharmaceutical industry, in order to sustain its products commercially, has begun to direct its interests towards the biomedical field. As the pharmaceutical industry needs to give scientific credibility to results of interest to it, the process of producing medical knowledge has become part of its negotiating arena.

Technological development and the production of scientific knowledge have been subjugated to economic interests - and medicine is no exception. As part of a conglomerate called the medical-industrial complex, the various negotiating points for scientific production make up the knowledge industry (CAMARGO JR., 2007).

As economic production came to depend on science as a value, the link between the pharmaceutical industry and the knowledge industry became a powerful mechanism supported by marketing strategies. Considering that the field of research is the main forum for validating empirical knowledge, funding research programs and producing scientific knowledge - according to their interests - has become a fundamental marketing strategy for the pharmaceutical industry.

Thus, the production of medical knowledge, scientifically legitimized through research, feeds the production of articles, guaranteeing both the circulation of knowledge and the sale of medicines. In this sense, the production of medical knowledge has become a production line supported by research, and information has become a commodity that leverages consumption.

An important part of the research, production and distribution of biomedical knowledge is under the control of private commercial interests. Considering the conflicts of interest and abuses of power, it is possible to gauge the seriousness of the effects of these distortions on public health policies, since, in medical interventions, knowledge plays a key role in the decision-making process (CAMARGO JR., 2007).

Captured by the capitalist system, the production of science goes through a process that puts science, scientists and the market at the same discussion table, where resources are defined. However, in addition to knowledge, other interests come into the negotiation. This means that all research issues are discussed in an arena that includes funding agencies, administrators, industries, publishers, directors of scientific institutions and suppliers. A structure termed by Knorr-Cetina (1981) as a "transepistemic arena" of negotiation.

Numerous problems arise from this context. Considering that what is at stake is the legitimization of knowledge, there is already a contradiction: although the reference point for truth lies in science, technical choices are not determined exclusively by scientists. The social construction of medical knowledge is thus tied to the industry's interests in legitimizing itself through science.

## 2.1 The Legitimization of Knowledge as a Marketing Strategy

The credibility of research in the area of medicines is conditioned by the demand for scientific legitimization of the use of the medicine, whose purpose, in biomedical logic, is preferably to combat specific diseases. This demand is anchored in the production of research that "demonstrates", in a "scientifically" appropriate way, the efficacy of the new drug in the specificity of its indication.

As a result of "this need" and with the aim of boosting sales, the industry has developed various forms of creative appropriation of research results as a strategy. This involves the use of techniques to skew results, such as expanding the user base of new drugs, or even creating new diseases or exaggerating the threat of harm - which, in English-language literature, is called *disease mongering* (MOYNIHAN & HENRY, 2006).

In his study on the process of constructing new dysfunctions or illnesses, Payer (2006) identified ten research manipulation tactics: 1- attributing to a normal function something wrong to be treated; 2- imputing suffering where none exists; 3- defining a large proportion of the population as susceptible to suffering from the illness; 4-

defining a condition of deficiency or imbalance; 5- giving a voice to *spin doctors,* communication specialists (who interpret results according to the interests at stake); 6- particularizing the approach to the subject; 7- exaggerating the benefits of treatment based on selective statistical data; 8- distorting the objective; 9- promoting technologies, treating them as "magically" risk-free; 10- taking a symptom, without any meaning, and making it sound like a sign of a serious illness (TIEFER, 2006).

Considering that the normal-pathological duality is structural in biomedical thinking (CANGUILHEM, 2006), the strategy consists of searching for a deviation from normal, the demarcation of which can support a demand for drug therapy. Due to inevitable socio-cultural components, there is a plasticity in the definition of "normality" - and therefore also of illness - which allows physiological phenomena to be transformed into "deviations"; in other words, when they are pathologized, they need to be treated.

Using the constructivist dimension of technical-scientific production as a reference, Hess (1995) defended, in his studies on class, gender, sex, race and ethnicity, the possibility of certain cultural aspects being re-signified by science and implanted socially. To designate this mechanism, the author used the metaphor of totemism (technototemism); and to explain the surprising ease with which society assimilates new knowledge and new technologies, he used the expression *strategies of circumvention.*

Perhaps it is from this perspective that the pharmaceutical industry, in order to introduce a certain substance onto the market, needs to associate knowledge with a socially assimilable reference. Insofar as sales are driven by the characterization of the product as scientific evidence, the mechanism is as described above: firstly, the focus of interest is on finding, from a biological conception, a consensual description of a state of nature; then, in order to characterize a deviation from this state, it is necessary to define a condition of abnormality; the next step is to invest in research aimed at correcting this presumed abnormality.

An example of this process in our society is described by Lexchin (2006), who tells how Pfizer transformed the action of Viagra® (sildenafil) - a treatment considered effective and safe for erectile dysfunction secondary to medical causes (diabetes, spinal diseases, etc.) - into a prescription for healthy men, with the aim of improving erectile performance, enabling them to maintain erection for longer.

Confined to the treatment of secondary causes, it would be a drug with very modest success due to the limited market. Pfizer's main motivation in sponsoring research into Viagra® was therefore to provide commercial backing for its launch. With the intention of transforming it into a product for widespread use among the male population, the criterion for success in the treatment of erectile dysfunction needed to be defined. This gave rise to the need to expand the perception of the prevalence of erectile dysfunction. The initial focus was on men over the age of 40, based on the assumption that they had significant concerns about erection. Finally, Viagra® was presented as an important treatment option for men with any degree of dysfunction, including rare or transient performance failures (LEXCHIN, 2006).

The reification of erection as the essence of male sexuality paved the way for the construction of the concept of male sexual dysfunction. In other words, data on male sexuality was captured and put at the service of the supposed ideal (or normal) condition. In the name of health, based on everyday findings, a powerful mechanism for intervening in life creates standardized forms of behaviour.

The scale of this medicalization process is such that the production of drugs in the area of sexuality is not aimed at the disease, but at increasing potency. Since the launch of Viagra® in 1998, more than 17 million prescriptions have been made for the treatment of erectile dysfunction. In 2001, Pfizer reported revenues of one and a half billion dollars (MOYNIHAN, 2003).

In an attempt to replicate the success achieved with the launch of Viagra® in female sexuality, the pharmaceutical industry is investing in a line of research that seeks out a new "reality": female sexual dysfunction. However, building a similar market among women requires a clear definition of the medical diagnosis, with measurable characteristics that give it clinical credibility, because the validation of biomedicine is done through epidemiological logic, that is, through representative samples provided by statistics.

Moynihan (2003) criticizes the sponsorship of research aimed at defining "female sexual dysfunction", the aim of which is to create needs and open up the market for other drugs. He gives as an example the publication of an article in JAMA in February 1999, in which the authors (linked to Pfizer) announced the 43% prevalence of sexual dysfunction in women aged between 18 and 59. After six months in the media, Pfizer announced that a new drug was being tested to treat female sexual disorders.

According to the author, the analysis of the data from this survey, carried out by sociologist Ed Laumann and colleagues, showed serious problems. Around 1,500 women were asked whether they had experienced any problems from a list of seven in the last few months of the previous year. The list included criteria for assessing sexuality, such as lack of sexual desire, anxiety about sexual *performance* and difficulties with lubrication. If the woman answered yes to one of the seven questions, she was included in the group characterized as sexual dysfunction.

As marketing strategies, this "scientific data" has been widely publicized in the media, with the following statement: "43% of women have dysfunction in one form or another, but not all of them have the most severe form". This is a process that seeks "public awareness of the problem", in other words, the acceptance of sexual dysfunction as a common and treatable illness (MOYNIHAN, 2003).

Pointing out controversies regarding the standardization of female physiological sexual responses and the process of medicalization of sexuality, Moynihan (2003) defends the importance of more rigorous monitoring of these research processes. For him, categorizing sexual difficulty as dysfunction is intended to induce doctors to prescribe drugs that "correct" sexual (dys)fungus.

Despite all this - with promotional *slogans* such as "Female Viagra arrives in Brazil" and "Now it's the women's turn" - a new product has already been launched on the Brazilian market with the promise of rescuing women's sexual pleasure. It's an intimate gel made up of arginine (an amino acid) and menthol (a substance that produces vasodilation) called Viatop-AM. Currently, the national laboratory Ativus Farmaceutica produces 11 (eleven) million units of products a year in two factories, located in Valinhos and Aguai, both in the interior of São Paulo. According to the company's managing director, Mascarenhas Marques Planeja, the investment will be concentrated on setting up a new production line for generic medicines: "We're going to launch 20 new products in this segment in 2008" (Source: Gazeta Mercantil de Sao Paulo, 12/12/2007).

With regard to the boundary between normal and pathological, we should refer to Canguilhem (2006): "If the normal does not have the rigidity of a collective coercive fact, but rather the flexibility of a norm that is transformed in its relationship with individual conditions, it is clear that the boundary between the normal and the pathological is imprecise. However, this does not lead us to the continuity of a normal and a pathological that are identical in essence [...], to a relativity of health and illness that is confusing enough to ignore where health ends and illness begins" (p. 135). This perspective points to the need for caution in relation to the concept of dysfunction. Because it is a misleading term, it mobilizes the boundary between health and illness in an excessive and dangerous way.

Another example of disease engineering was developed by the Lilly laboratory in the construction of bipolar disorder. Through a *website* called the *Bipolar Help Center* (http://www.bipolarhelpcenter.com/resources/mdq.jsp), Lilly implemented a questionnaire on bipolar disorder. At the same time, a TV ad warned of the possibility of psychiatric illness, inducing viewers to take the test and show it to their doctor. This with the argument that diagnosis is the first step to treating bipolar disorder (HEALY, 2006).

This announcement came in 2002, shortly after the antipsychotic olanzepine (Zyprexa®), launched by the pharmaceutical company Lilly, was licensed to treat mania. The laboratory quickly invested in research to link the drug to mood stabilization. Currently, interest is focused on building the diagnosis of bipolar disorder in American children. Without traditional diagnostic criteria, several publications have appeared on the subject: the book *The Bipolar Child* (Papoulos, 2000) and the article "Young and Bipolar", published in the American edition of TIME magazine (August 2002), among others (HEALY, 2006).

According to Healy (2006), this "awareness" of the need for mood stabilization has been surprising. For him, even if we only consider adults, there is already the potential to create an "epidemic" of bipolar disorder, because people are being diagnosed on the basis of non-objective operational criteria.

Today, with the argument that teachers can help diagnose attention deficit hyperactivity disorder, the industry has developed a new mechanism to infiltrate schools. As part of the industry's promotional marketing strategies, while teachers are trained to identify the disease and the need for medication, doctors are encouraged to prescribe and monitor therapeutic results (PHILLIPS, 2006).

## 2.2 Research and Publications: as Strategies in the Promotion of Medicines

A close relationship between research and scientific production fuels the production of articles, the dissemination of knowledge and the sale of medicines. It involves the interests of the pharmaceutical industry in funding research, the results of which become scientific knowledge to be published and disseminated. This dynamic is characterized as a powerful link between the pharmaceutical industry and the knowledge industry. With a concentrated interest in the publication and propagation of medical knowledge, the pharmaceutical industry - without prioritizing quality - invests in the quantity of publications. Thus, the production of medical knowledge has become a line of production sustained by research.

The need to give credibility to results of economic interest has led the pharmaceutical industry to invest in pseudo-research. Despite the appearance of real research, its aim is not to produce new knowledge. These studies are actually marketing strategies, with deliberately biased methodology to strengthen the commercial position of a particular drug, with results that "prove" what is being said by propagandists.

Numerous "multicenter studies" carry out clinical trials involving substances with proven efficacy and which are well-established on the market; their sole aim is to corroborate them so that they can be presented to new markets. In general, their results are disseminated in a big way, in places where there are opinion formers and doctors in training - as is the case with university hospitals.

Conceived as the producer of absolute truths, science gives knowledge the category of myth. This resonates with the susceptibility of doctors to assimilate any information from the scientific world as true. It is in this context of pre-established ideas, in which doctors refrain from critically analyzing the results, that the pharmaceutical industry emerges as a funder of research and appropriates the possibility of directing interests in the biomedical area.

By encouraging the productivity of knowledge, the industry plays on the idea of irremediable technological progress. In this way, it justifies the huge volume of publications, producing in doctors - whose recognition depends on keeping up to date - the unsettling feeling of being permanently short of this possibility (CAMARGO JR., 2003).

In its symbolic meaning, knowledge represents capital, and this value encourages doctors to appropriate it (BOURDIEU, 2005). In order to keep up to date, doctors follow the conclusions of specialist authors on research reports, whose scientific evidence feeds the medical literature. If medical books are based on these results, it is essential that these reports are absolutely impartial.

In this sense, there are already studies that point to the propensity of industry-sponsored researchers to favor the company's products. The biased nature of trials can be seen in the simple suppression of negative results, or when the researcher praises a drug whose results do not justify any enthusiasm. This bias can also be built into the research design, as in the case of placebo-controlled clinical trials (inert pill). This means that the drug is being compared to nothing; and that, when compared to other drugs on the market, they may actually prove to be less effective than when compared to placebos. There are trials to study drugs aimed at treating older people, whose tests are carried out on young people. In other cases, the new drug is compared with an old drug given at an excessively low dose (ANGELL, 2007).

In most industry-sponsored clinical trials to test new drugs or procedures, the protocols are drawn up by the sponsor and the data collected is sent in its raw state to be analyzed by the sponsor. This means that the participation of doctors in research does not go beyond including patients and carrying out the procedures laid out in a standardized protocol (GUIMARAES, 2007).

In a recent study, the author (2007) shows that the situation becomes even more complicated when it comes to the qualification of published articles. The merit and/or relevance of scientific contributions are considered based on a category called "impact", indicated by the number of times the article is cited in indexed journals. This "impact" is strongly influenced by the way in which the research was organized: 1- large networks of researchers with the potential to attract patients who submit to standardized protocols; 2- remuneration for researchers per patient attracted; 3- no guarantee of ethical research standards. In the cases analyzed by Guimaraes (2007), it is possible (probable, according to the author) that the participation of national authors in the articles in question was negligible; nevertheless, they will receive formal credit for their authorship, recognized by the bodies that evaluate research production in the country (CAPES, CNPQ, state research support foundations). This represents a potential bias in the mechanisms for establishing academic merit towards purely commercial interests, an aspect which, incidentally, Brazilian science has not yet paid attention to (GUIMARAES, 2007).

Despite all this, in relation to Brazil, Guimaraes (2007) argues that the funding of clinical trials by industry or other external institutions should not be discouraged or restricted, as long as ethical standards and republican practices of remuneration per patient are guaranteed.

An example of this process is the case of gabapentin (Neurotin®): a drug approved by the FDA in 1994 to treat only epileptic seizures not controlled by other drugs. In order to expand the market, Parke-Davis devised a plan called the "advertising strategy" to get doctors to prescribe Neurotin® for unapproved uses. The US government took the company to court for this violation. In 2004, Pfizer (which incorporated Parke-Davis in 2000) admitted its responsibility for violating federal regulations in the promotion of gabapentin, ending the case through a settlement with the government.

Subsequently, on the basis of the *Freedom of Information Act,* a group of researchers obtained access to company documents submitted to the courts (ANGELL, 2007). By analyzing these documents, Steinman, Bero, Chren and Landerfeld (2006) identified three specific groups of doctors as the target of the laboratory's marketing interests: 1- a group of doctors selected on the basis of the dollar/prescription ratio; 2- a key group made up of doctors with influential power (program exhibitors); 3- a group made up of leaders, identified by their role in local medical associations.

In order to convey the idea of involvement in medical practice, Parke-Davis allocated specific budget to "resident programs": educational methods; payment to medical lecturers; creation of advisory boards; promotion of consultant meetings; as well as research and publication strategies. The analysis of internal documentation showed the enormous extent of the laboratory's marketing activities, far beyond the open advertising they pointed to as the tip of the iceberg. Most of the activities (and resources) take place as covert advertising, including all the strategies described above (STEINMAN; BERO; CHREN; LANDERFELD, 2006).

According to Angell (2007), based on the results of the research funded by the laboratory, articles would be written for specialized publications. Medical education companies were hired to write the articles and find "authors" to sign them. One of them, for example, received US$12,000 for each of the 12 journal articles it prepared, and paid academic "authors" US$1,000 per subscription. In one of the reports sent to Parke-Davis, the company signaled that it was having trouble finding anyone to sign, and wrote: "Author interested, still playing hide and seek by phone" And then, in capital letters: "[OUR FIRM] HAS THE TEXT READY, WE JUST NEED AN AUTHOR" (p. 174).

To the extent that the interest in funding research and interfering in its results is related to the pharmaceutical industry's marketing strategies, resources end up being directed towards trials that give satisfactory results, i.e. that publicize the laboratory and increase profits. Despite the efforts to keep the real interests at stake veiled, the biased targeting of resources reveals important contradictions, i.e. although the industry's discourse announces collaboration in the production of medical knowledge, this collaboration is not committed to Public Health. This means that the research being carried out does not, strictly speaking, have a research objective; it is therefore pseudo-research.

Although the target consumer is the end consumer, the pharmaceutical industry makes a specific investment in medical staff. With enormous economic power, it offers a wide variety of incentives: promotion of events, travel expenses, hotels, gifts, books and advertising leaflets, etc. The discourse of prioritizing the health and safety of consumers actually conceals the main objective: to promote the sale of medicines.

The industry representative uses the issue of medical rationality to manipulate; and he touches on the points where the doctor is vulnerable. By announcing a series of new drugs, he corroborates the idea of frequent changes in medical knowledge. However, a closer look shows that the majority of so-called pharmacological innovations actually derive from minor modifications to existing products or simply patent renewals. If science is manipulated in this way, it shows us the importance of developing a critical capacity not only for research, but also for the quality of the knowledge disseminated (CAMARGO JR., 2007).

Another aspect pointed out by Knorr-Cetina (1981) is the unequal struggle between agents with different capital endowments; an inequality that compromises the ability both to resist the imposition of products and to appropriate the results of scientific work. For peripheral countries, this creates serious problems within the process of negotiating the production of knowledge: difficulty in accessing both the content and the results of tests. With a dynamic conditioned to payment, the countries of Africa, for example, end up being systematically excluded from ventures related to scientific production, even though important parts of the research have been carried out on their territory, with their population.

It is generally agreed that commercial interests should not influence medical decisions in favor of the patient. Given the ineffectiveness of efforts to manage these conflicts, new strategies need to be implemented: not neglecting strict regulation; making a strict separation between commercial and scientific activities; as well as a thorough re-evaluation of the interaction between medical professionals, professional organizations and industry.

In Brazil, this interaction can be exemplified by the periodic reformulation of the antiretroviral therapy (ART) consensus for the treatment of HIV-infected people, with two main objectives: to guide the Ministry of Health in the purchase and distribution of drugs and to assist doctors in the management of HIV-positive people, in accordance with the latest scientific evidence.

In 1996, the Ministry of Health's National STD and AIDS Coordination, advised by AIDS treatment specialists, formulated the first ART consensus to guide doctors across the country. Since then, the advisory committee has periodically evaluated the inclusion of new drugs and defined new recommendations. With 180,000 patients receiving antiretroviral drugs, the new therapeutic consensus for adults with AIDS was released by the Ministry of Health in October 2007.

This process is an example of how the knowledge needed for health actions can be publicly appropriated; in a way that is much less subject to interference from commercial interests and more in line with the health demands of the population.

## 3 Power/Knowledge: An Inseparable Link

This study analyzes contemporary power relations in order to understand the micropolitical dimension of the biomedical knowledge production process. It does so within a dynamic that articulates epistemological aspects with economic interests. Pointed out by Foucault in *Microphysics of Power,* this micropolitics functions, within society, as a fine network whose configuration results from a set of strategic positions of power relations. Against the backdrop of a biopolitical project, it produces realities such as conceptions of health, consumption of medicines and technologies, etc. (FOUCAULT, 1995).

The previous topic dealt with the issue of knowledge production in the context of a macro-political system in which the dominant power (represented by the pharmaceutical industry) articulates with the knowledge industry in order to direct interests. Through marketing strategies (power techniques), the contemporary construction of biomedical knowledge is conditioned to the same logic as the capitalist production and distribution of merchandise.

In this sense, considering society's force field, medicine is limited by a power that is outside the specifically medical ambit. As well as contradicting the supposed social omnipotence of medicine, this points to a process of colonization of the medical profession. As a result of the linking of industry interests to the symbolic meaning attributed to health within society, the medical discourse, as the foundation of the Contemporary Clinic, has come to be used as a power strategy (CAMARGO Jr., 1995, p. 19).

In Foucault's logic, it is in the way the "power-knowledge" relationship (ideological power) is articulated that the current political system (political power) (historically) bases its configuration of power; in other words, discourse and power. To the extent that knowledge is tied to economic interests, scientific production itself functions as an instrument of power, and medical discourse is exploited by the pharmaceutical industry as a "power technique".

Although there is marketing with the aim of consumption, specifically aimed at the population, it should be emphasized that the central point of this dynamic is to interfere in the prescriptive practices of doctors. Strategically manipulated through (colonizing) power techniques, the doctor ends up functioning as the link in a chain that connects the knowledge industry to guaranteed sales of pharmaceutical products. This mechanism feeds and closes the cycle of the industries' economic power: on the one hand, the "colonized" medical profession, and on the other, the "hyper-medicalized" society.

In addition to interfering in the process of producing and applying medical knowledge, these strategies jeopardize the evaluation of the efficacy of medicines, since they involve the credibility criteria attributed to knowledge that is presented as new and likely to replace current practices. They touch on critical points in a process whose complexity involves doctors' conceptions of the construction of knowledge, since doctors' belief in the scientificity of knowledge and the biomedical logic of its application is used by the industry in favor of its manipulation interests (CAMARGO, 2003).

However, it is important to note that, for Foucault (1997), there is no separation between knowledge on the one hand and society on the other; nor between science on the one hand and the state on the other. No knowledge is formed outside a context of power, just as no power is exercised without appropriating knowledge. However, it is not a question of determining how power subordinates knowledge, imposing content and ideological limitations on it. The way society functions rests on a system of power that defines what should be constituted as knowledge (FOUCAULT, 1997).

When Foucault says that "the body is a biopolitical reality and medicine is a biopolitical strategy" (FOUCAULT, 1995, p. 80), he is referring to a micropolitical dynamic in whose configuration of power the very biology of the individual - the body and life - is the main part of the system of power, transforming the production of subjectivity into the focus of global hegemony. It is in this sense that Foucault inaugurates a new conception of power, saying that power has no pre-defined place or form; there are conformations of power, always according to the forces at play.

By considering the power/knowledge relationship as inseparable, Foucault situates the power of medical discourse in the symbolic context of the contemporary biopolitical project - which, understood as relations of force, places the production of medical knowledge in the hands of the pharmaceutical industry (FOUCAULT, 1979).

Directed by economic power, its political rationale translates into the ethical-political-scientific appropriation of the body (biopolitical reality) and of life (with medicine as a strategy) by contemporary consumer societies. In the cultural imagination, this dimension is exploited biopolitically to the exact extent that medicine has disease as its object and that, in practice, the "sick biological body" needs to be treated (GOOD, 1999).

Considering the biological foundation as a strategic point of articulation between medical knowledge and market expectations, this study seeks to understand, on the continent of contemporary biopolitics, how the medical style of thinking (FLECK, 1979) is used by the industry as a strategic mechanism of power.

### 3.1 Power in Foucault's conception

The concept of power developed by Foucault contrasts with the classical concept constructed by Hobbes (2004) with the idea of Sovereign Power: centralized, localized and related to the idea of total domination by the sovereign. In this way, power transcends man. In Foucault's conception, power has no place, nor is it something that is possessed; it is a relationship of forces. The philosophical key to understanding power in this way is to think of it as the immanent exercise of each force in its field of forms. Power, understood as relations of power or relations of forces, goes through the ages with different configurations, representations and strategic power techniques (DELEUZE, 1998).

The representation of power should not be confused with the configuration of power. In fact, the "place" instituted as a representation of power strategically "represents" the historically configured power. Medieval society saw a configuration of power with two types of power in dispute: political power (of the State), exercised through physical force, by means of weapons; and spiritual power (of the Church), through religious discourse, with threats of punishment or promises of ultra-terrestrial rewards (power/knowledge) (BOBBIO, 1986).

In Modernity, the configuration of power was represented by the Modern State, which, in its articulation of power and knowledge, was based on laws - political and legal sovereignty. Then, under the aegis of the concept of national sovereignty, the nation-state was established, which brought the idea of the people of a nation into its articulation of power/knowledge (HARDT and NEGRI, 2001).

With the evolution of capitalism, bourgeois ideology - previously dominantly based on legal principles - reinforced itself as the holder of power/knowledge, legitimized by technical-scientific knowledge. This moment historically marked the appropriation of science by capital and the state, giving rise to a new configuration of power: science became an instrument of the mechanisms of power (HARDT and NEGRI, 2001).

According to Bobbio, there are three types of canonical power: economic, ideological and political, which act simultaneously in society. Economic power is in the hands of those who own the means of production; ideological power is based on knowledge and doctrines; and political power is the state, which has the right to use force (BOBBIO, 1986, p. 81).

In the contemporary configuration of power - the process of globalization - the force of economic power is exercised in a dominant way in relation to the state (political power). In Foucault's logic, it is in the form of the articulation of the "power-knowledge" relationship (ideological power) that the current political system (political power) is based.

(historically) its configuration of power; in other words, it is a dynamic in which discourse (knowledge) functions as a power strategy.

## 3.2 Biopower and Biopolitics: from the Disciplinary Society to the Control Society

Historically, Biopower (disciplinary) succeeded Sovereign Power. As a result of the accumulation of capital, a new social reality emerged: death left the ambit of power and life became its object. In sovereign power, both life and death (of subjects) were part of the political field. In disciplinary power, the model is individualization - Bentham's panoptism[1] . Visibility, previously located in the "subject of power" (the sovereign), shifts to the subjected individual, "subject to power".

In Biopower, as a reality of contemporary civilization, what is at stake is the production and reproduction of life. The strategic technique is to involve life completely and manage it. Biopower, as a technique for making people live, takes two main forms: Discipline and Biopolitics (Power of Control) (PALBERT, 2003, p. 57).

In disciplinary power, discipline is directed at the body, because it is in action that discipline is exercised. Power is combined with knowledge, and knowledge becomes a function of power. Power wants docile and productive bodies; knowledge helps to extract from each body what power needs. In short, discipline is a set of techniques that targets individuals in their singularities (FOUCAULT, 1995, p. 105-107).

The dominant medical discourse arose from the political, economic and social situation in Europe at the end of the 18th century. Due to the configuration of power in force, medicine was exercised through disciplinary techniques, with the aim of normalizing individuals. Here, Biopower emerged, the name given by Foucault (1995) to the disciplinary power of Medicine.

Medical practices and their medicalizing devices, in search of the normal individual, have become consumer goods. The expansion of Biopower reached its peak in the mid-20th century with the installation of the disciplinary model in all

[1] At the end of the 18th century, Jeremy Bentham, an English jurist, designed the panopticon, an architectural model of a circular prison with a central tower; from there, a guard permanently watches over the prisoners. Foucault was inspired by panopticism to study disciplinary power ("The eye of power". In: *Microphysics of Power*. Jean-Pierre Barou interviews Foucault).

social institutions, such as hospitals, schools, universities, prisons, etc. Once the interdependence between the hospital and anatomo-clinical knowledge had been established, the hospital became a place of healing and teaching; articulating discipline and knowledge.

This disciplinary dimension of medicine acts as an important instrument of power in the force field of contemporary society. Allied to education and the legal system, it determines their functioning and interferes in the processes of constructing social realities. Disciplinary power masks social conflicts as "medical problems" and works towards normalization (of docile bodies) through medical practices.

Medicalizing power is exercised through a relationship of domination and expropriation of knowledge. With enormous weight in society, conceptions of health determine ways of being in the world. Exploited by the media, life has become a dangerous thing; existential aspects have been transformed into illness, creating an imperative need for permanent protection.

To the extent that the very biology of the individual became central to the system of power, Biopower, associated with scientific knowledge, took the form of scrutiny, creating a new social structure. As part of a billion-dollar context of planetary consumption, the process of medicalization is supported by a theoretical framework - biomedical knowledge - which is given the status of Science (CAMARGO, 1995).

In his book *Normal and Pathological*, Canguilhem (2006) re-reads the scientific clinic *and* studies the organism's ability to define norms in relation to the world. Foucault opposes this idea by saying that the organism does not produce norms. It is the norms that are imposed by the social sphere in order to produce "norms". In this sense, the categories of normal, abnormal and pathological are part of a project of Normalization - a project of Medical Modelling (BIRMAN, 2005).

In modern thinking, Biopolitics was just a naming system by definition. *Bios:* life. *Polis:* city (politics). In the 1970s, with the transition from classic capitalism to integrated world capitalism, a new economic discourse emerged - with a neoliberal tendency - accompanied by enormous technological advances. Political and social changes had major repercussions in the medical field, including on the traditional foundations of medical practice and discourse.

Coinciding with neoliberalism, a new language game has given the concept of Biopolitics a new meaning. A constituent part of Foucault's work (1977), Biopolitics was conceived as a dimension of Biopower in "Security, Territory, Population" (BIRMAN, 2005). Foucault coined the term "biopolitics" to designate one of the ways in which power is exercised over life, a political power focused on biological processes. The object of power is the population, the global mass. "Biopolitics" has come to designate the mechanisms for using the body and life, making power/knowledge an agent for transforming human life, always under the explicit domination of power (PAL PELBART, 2003).

With Biopolitics, a new conception of life is at stake. A new place is assigned to life. A new form of control over the body comes into existence in the social context, related to the production of wealth (capitalism) and linked to the population's quality of life. Thus, in the name of wealth, in the name of the population's quality of life, a new way of controlling individuals emerges - from the control of bodies in the social space and through instrumentalization - medicalization (BIRMAN, 2005).

Biopower refers to a situation in which what is directly at stake in power is the production and reproduction of life itself. According to Hardt and Negri (2001), Foucault's work prepared the ground for a historical transition of biopower: from the disciplinary society to the control society, bringing about a new biopolitical configuration.

Hardt and Negri (2001), in their book *Imperia,* analyze this biopolitical transition, outlining the main differences in the contemporary configuration of Biopower. For them, the social command of disciplinary society is carried out through disciplinary institutions, producing and regulating customs, habits and productive practices whose obedience is sustained by logical explanations - parameters and limits of thought and practice - appropriate to the "reason" of discipline, which sanction and prescribe normal and/or deviant behavior (HARDT, NEGRI, 2001).

In the society of control, command mechanisms are immanent in the social field. Regardless of the meaning of life and the desire for creation, power is exercised, producing a state of alienation. The brain is organized through communication systems and information networks, and bodies are subjected to monitored activities and welfare systems. It is therefore characterized by the intensification and synthesis of the mechanisms of normalization and disciplinarization; but, unlike discipline, by acting within daily practices, through flexible and fluctuating networks, it goes beyond social institutions (HARDT, NEGRI, 2001).

In this sense, the contemporary biopolitical project is exercised through a Biopower that regulates social life from the inside, monitoring, interpreting, absorbing and rearticulating. To the extent that it has become an integral and vital function, embraced and reactivated by everyone, freely and spontaneously, power has effectively acquired total command over the lives of the population. As Foucault said, "life has now become an object of power" (HARDT and NEGRI, 2001).

In disciplinary society, the relationship between power and the individual remained stable: the effect of biopolitical technology was still partial and the disciplinary invasion of power corresponded to the individual's resistance. At the pace of productive practices and productive socialization, the process of disciplinarization fixed individuals in institutions, but did not manage to consume them completely, it did not permeate the consciousness and body of individuals in an integral way (HARDT, NEGRI, 2001).

To the extent that technologies have recognized society as the realm of biopower, it has become entirely biopolitical; the entire social body has been embraced by the machinery of power and developed into its virtualities. It is a society that reacts as a single body, subjected to a power that acts on the totality of social relations and that reaches into the "ganglia" of the social structure and extends deep into the consciousness and bodies of the population (HARDT, NEGRI, 2001).

Therefore, in this transition from disciplinary society to the society of control, it can be said that capitalism has finally achieved a mutual relationship with social forces, which it has always sought throughout its development. If, however, subordinations are understood in terms of the social *bios* itself, i.e. beyond the economic or social dimensions of society, the totalitarian image of capitalist development is dispelled. For Hardt and Negri (2001), this means that Foucault constructed a paradox of power, because by unifying and involving all the elements of social life, power loses its ability to mediate different social forces, revealing a new context of maximum plurality and unavoidable singularization.

Despite this configuration of power, which has contemporary biopolitics as its backdrop, this study continues in its task of analyzing, in the current context, the dominant forces in the composition of the medical knowledge production process. In this vein, the question arises of what is more important, the organ or the function of the organ. This question is answered by Foucault, who says that it is through the function of the organ that Biopolitics is inserted. For him, the population to be "normalized" is the object, in itself, of Biopolitics (BIRMAN, 2005).

# 4 The Epistemic Dimension in the Configuration of Medical Power-Knowledge

As Foucault teaches, through the articulation of power/knowledge, dominant knowledge subordinates other knowledge, creating new symbolic representations of power. It is in this sense that the style of medical thought (FLECK, 1979) offers, in its very foundation, a condition conducive to exploitation by the mechanisms of power: the technical-scientific foundations of medical thought.

To the extent that this "epistemological obstacle" is manipulated and used in the process of the social construction of knowledge, it is medicine itself, the style of medical thinking, that becomes vulnerable to the techniques of the dominant powers. This, in society's field of forces, is reflected in the disputes that exist in power relations, calling into question the validity of scientifically produced knowledge.

In his epistemological study, Fleck (1979) philosophically substantiates the nature of the scientific process, saying that truth in science is defined according to a particular style of thinking within a collective of thought. For the author, style of thought refers to a "definite construal of thought" (p. 64), or rather, a totalizing intellectual disposition, which determines a particular way of thinking, seeing and acting. The collective of thought refers to an intellectual community whose way of thinking is stabilized through the mutual interaction of ideas.

In this conception, there is no absolute truth; the conception of truth is not a subjective question. The "true" corresponds to a singular solution, which is the result of a particular way of thinking, whether intersubjective or collective. Therefore, the inclusion of a "truth" in a collective way of thinking is imposed by the process of socialization; and it can change according to time and culture (FLECK, 1979, p. 155-157).

Incorporating Fleck's philosophical concepts as the theoretical underpinning of this study, it can be said that, in the process of contemporary production of medical knowledge, "true" knowledge emerges from the collective of medical thought (medical intellectual community), whose attribution of truth depends on collective acceptance and is directly related to the style of medical thought.

With science as a structuring element of Western culture, the production of medical knowledge involves medical rationality itself and the concept of evidence. If the scientific presupposition of medicine lies in evidence, the key to safe knowledge lies in the objectivity of the evidence itself. However, through the mechanisms of manipulation of the dominant power, philosophically validating what science presents as a scientific construction requires a critical analysis of the nature of the methods by which evidence was arrived at.

From this perspective, it should be borne in mind that when epidemiological investigations are carried out using inductive probabilistic methods, the phenomena revealed in clinical analysis are presented in a statistically quantified form, which makes data analysis more difficult. Because it is a mathematical form, the problem is that the representation of the phenomenon tested goes beyond the condition of probability and takes on a causal dimension. Under the tutelage of the interests of pharmaceutical laboratories, the pharmacopoeia of risk potential reduction was born out of this clinical/epidemiologic device.

Boaventura (2005) helps us understand this context when he says that the economy has overflowed into the social sphere and political debate has been replaced by economic debate. This is a field of forces characterized by a style of thought conditioned by economic rhetoric. Subjected to an articulation between epistemology and the pharmaceutical market, medical therapy may be distancing itself from a place that should be absolutely ethical.

Here we can see a contemporary relativism, increasingly evident in the scientific world, which epistemologically translates into the difficulty of identifying ethically, aesthetically and politically defensible principles.

### 4.1 - Medical Discourse: A Style of Thinking

The technical-scientific medical discourse emerged on the threshold of modernity from a rupture in medical knowledge, fundamentally transforming the process of constructing knowledge. The incorporation of anatomy into medical knowledge meant the birth of a medicine of the body, of injuries and illnesses. This outlined a new epistemological field: the search for the essence of illness, based on the empirical examination of injuries. A central category of medical knowledge and practice, illness was affirmed as the result of a cause to be identified by characterizing the injury; and therapeutic indication came to depend on the ability to reach the cause (FOUCAULT, 1998).

Medical knowledge, therefore, as well as being based on the consensual way in which medical practice is carried out, has as its unstated support a set of representations that form the backbone of "medical science". It is a kind of "theory of diseases", which functions as a medical doctrine, saying that diseases affirm their concrete existence through injuries, announced by a set of signs and symptoms. Diseases must be sought out in the heart of the organism and combated through therapeutic, medicinal or surgical intervention (CAMARGO Jr., 2003).

For Canguilhem (2006), however, medicine should not be considered a science per se, but "a technique for establishing and restoring the normal, which cannot be entirely reduced to simple knowledge" (p. 6-7). In this sense, the production of medical knowledge is dominated by biology and based on a scientific "ideology" because, despite the efforts of scientific rationalization, the essence of medicine remains clinical and therapeutic. This means that, because of the need to find the biological mechanism of disease, determinism demands the essence of the cause, with reductionism as the dominant model in the construction of knowledge. According to the author:

> The ambition to make pathology and, consequently, therapeutics fully scientific [...] would only make sense if it were possible to give a purely objective definition of normal as de facto; and if, furthermore, it were possible to translate any difference between the normal and pathological states in terms of quantity, because only quantity can account for both homogenization and variation. (CANGUILHEM, 2006, p. 26)

Reaffirming his thoughts on the construction of medical knowledge, the author quotes Comte to defend the independence of theoretical biology from medicine and therapeutics (p. 65). And he recognizes Claude Bernard's innovative authority in believing in the omnipotence of technique, based on medical science (p. 53). Common to both authors is the concept of technique as the application of a science and the fundamental positivist idea: to know in order to act. Physiology must explain pathology in order to lay the foundations for therapy. Ultimately, for both, the logical procedure starts from experimental physiological knowledge to medical technique (p. 64).

In view of these aspects, the epistemic dimension of medicine is permeated by two conflicting tendencies: that of certainties, where the logic is deterministic, i.e. there is causality; and that of probabilities: interpreted and used (strategic manipulation of results) as if it were deterministic. The two tendencies are not opposed, but are part of different disciplinary fields. The problem is that, due to rationality, the study of causes ends up favoring deterministic logic, putting experience on one side and science/technology on the other.

Epistemic authority carries significant weight in the medical profession, but, according to Weisz (2002), when it comes to producing a statement, the idea of objectivity eliminates human agency. In medicine, this acts as an obstacle because, to the extent that the knowledge considered true is that which is independent of human agency, its subjective dimension is eliminated from medical practice. It is because of this that probability takes the lead in the search for regularity: to work with random elements, filter out noise signals from variability and observe their effects with statistical techniques.

Although there are two possible approaches to the production of medical knowledge - deterministic and probabilistic - what happens in practice is that the probabilistic models end up being captured by the deterministic ones. Although probability is not deterministic, when, for example, studies show that smoking causes lung cancer in 13% of cases, probabilistic data is assimilated as determinant and, as a result, transformed into a risk factor.

For philosopher Ian Hacking, probability is the relationship between hypothesis and evidence. This hides the explanation of probability and places the concept of evidence as a precondition of probability. On the other hand, according to the author, for modern epistemologists, the concept of evidence depends on the stabilization of the concept of induction. Although the concept of "inductive evidence" is imprecise, some philosophers use it to exclude the evidence attributed by the senses (HACKING, 1975).

Modern epistemology considers the internal evidence of things to be the foundation of evidence, which needs to be contextualized before the experimental method. In this sense, testing means giving new "inductive evidence" to the hypothesis, in other words, rationally verifying the relevance of the hypothesis. The philosophers' ambiguity regarding "inductive evidence" has, on the one hand, evidence "induced" by the generalization of the law of nature, gained from particular observation; on the other hand, the "induction" of evidence will always be from one particular piece of evidence (which emerged first) to another particular piece of evidence (HACKING, 1975).

The probability is considered significant when it reaches a value lower than a proportion arbitrarily chosen to define the probability of a random association. Although the disciplinary autonomy of epidemiology has been reinforced by the computer, despite the progressive improvement of the determination of mathematical significance, the logic of statistical inference has not changed.

An important epistemological break, the process of association with statistics meant that epidemiology consolidated its epistemological prestige. By technically assimilating quantitative methods, it ceased to be a discipline focused solely on describing epidemics. By analyzing the causes of disease, epidemiological research became the key to validating knowledge about disease theory.

As a branch of Public Health, epidemiology began to use statistics as a tool. It acquired the ability to produce clinical evidence and, as a result, many researchers directed their studies towards identifying risk factors. In this way, it can be said that Evidence-Based Medicine was born out of its articulation with Clinical Epidemiology.

Therefore, it is from epidemiology that diseases emerge as a theoretical construct, in whose "theoretical body", as in the clinic, the disease is seen as a natural entity with no history. This means that, despite its methodological prestige in the production of knowledge, epidemiology is subordinate to biological knowledge and the biological sciences. As part of contemporary medical rationality, epidemiological evidence is subject to the same scientific ideology (CAMARGO Jr., 2003).

In epidemiology, causal relationships are established by observing various population groups, named according to the presence or absence of causes of disease. The resulting tabulation is analyzed using statistically significant associations between factors and effects. It was in this context of "symbiosis" between epidemiology and clinical medicine, in which one depends on the other for the elaboration of its objects, that the pharmaceutical industry began to exploit the epistemological model of biomedicine in order to meet market interests (CAMARGO JR., 2003).

Epidemiology works with probabilities using the inductive method in order to identify diseases. It is essential to the clinic, as it allows for the generalization necessary to place medicine within the natural sciences. On the other hand, however, the clinical paradigm is "indicative" (GINZBURG, 1989); in other words, instead of generalizing, it individualizes based on the reading of signs. This means that medical practice, being extremely dependent on the individual experience of the doctor, cannot be reduced to the analytical criteria of conventional scientific logic. As a result, in order to acquire scientific legitimacy, medicine needed to invoke science, or rather, it needed to incorporate the scientific model in order to develop (CAMARGO Jr., 2003). In this dynamic, the epistemological aspects that underpin medical intervention are used strategically by the industry to study the causes of illnesses and their respective treatments. In line with its commercial interests, the industry uses the medical discourse itself and its foundations to interfere strategically in the process of social construction of medical knowledge; in other words, the techniques of power are based on characteristics extracted from the very logic of medical thought (style of medical thought).

### 4.2 Probabilistic Risk Comprehension: An Extrapolation of Power Techniques

Strengthening the interests of industry, there is a socially installed research culture that makes science function as a place of power. In the wake of this ideology, research funding has become a vital link between knowledge production and pharmaceutical development. This means that, at every stage of the process of producing and disseminating medical knowledge, as well as in its translation into medical practice, there is an amalgam between the market and research. In this configuration, disease is no longer just an epidemiological event, but also a market event (GREENE, 2007).

When presenting and launching new drugs, the marketing strategies (power techniques) of pharmaceutical laboratories rely on two main rhetorical arguments. Firstly, the drug must be a product of scientific research. Secondly, it has to be intended to fight disease.

As for the requirement of scientific legitimacy, clinical trials need to demonstrate scientifically, in an appropriate manner, that the drug fulfills its advertised therapeutic efficacy. At the same time, the industry has developed ways of creatively appropriating research results out of the "need" to boost sales. As part of final reports, these "results" are transformed into rhetorical arguments and used as a marketing strategy to present new drugs to the market.

The "production of disease" has become an important commercial strategy, as it convinces the population of the need for medical intervention. This mechanism involves two serious and complex issues: it pathologizes physiological conditions and expands the concept of disease to mild or pre-symptomatic forms, such as the characterization of "high cholesterol" as a disease. Diagnosed through laboratory tests, this risk factor, now classified as a disease, indicates the need for medication (MOYNIHAN and HENRY, 2006).

Angell (2007), when addressing the power of pharmaceutical laboratories to influence the production of medical knowledge, states that "the industry's influence on medical research is clearly aimed at biasing data to ensure that their drugs perform well". In view of the funding of research as a strategy for interfering in its results, it is very worrying that pharmaceutical laboratories are increasingly investing in clinical tests aimed at the causes of diseases and their respective treatments (ANGELL, 2007).

It should be noted, however, that the initial stages of drug development are based on market potential. Furthermore, due to their involvement in funding clinical trials, shareholders have increasingly become as responsible for research as scientists and regulators (GREENE, 2007).

For Angell (2007), although the rhetoric of the pharmaceutical industry is based on Research and Development - for the sake of science - this does not correspond to reality. Firstly, because investment in R&D, when compared to expenditure on marketing and administration, is a tiny part of the company's budget (even smaller than profits). Despite the fact that the pharmaceutical industry is the most profitable in the United States, the price charged for drugs bears little relation to production costs. This means that even if the budget were to be cut drastically, this would not threaten R&D activities in any way (ANGELL, 2007).

Secondly, because the pharmaceutical industry is not particularly innovative. Few major drugs have been launched on the market in recent years. The products presented as "new" are, for the most part, "copycat drugs" whose production targets a slice of an already consolidated market. For example, there are six cholesterol-lowering "statins" on the market: Mevacor®, Lipitor®, Zocor®, Pravacol®, Lescol® and, most recently, Crestor®, all variants of the first (ANGELL, 2007).

Thirdly, the pharmaceutical industry is totally dependent on government-granted monopolies - approved by the *Food and Drug Administration* (FDA)[2] , in the form of patents and exclusive marketing rights. As a result, the industry has been extremely creative - and aggressive - in inventing ways to extend monopoly rights and patents; as well as pouring money into legal maneuvers. Although they are indeed profitable, instead of prioritizing investment in innovative drugs and price moderation, they are investing heavily in marketing and lobbying to prevent the government from adopting any form of price regulation (ANGELL, 2007).

In 1971, the data from a study evaluating 228 companies in Brazil, which represented 50% of the companies established in the country, and which had 81% of the turnover, led CEME to suggest "a massive concentration of *know-how* and resources in the hands of extra-national groups, This trend towards the incorporation of national companies into multinationals was confirmed by the transfer of control of 43 companies in the period 1958-1973. Accompanied by a loss of competitiveness,

[2] FDA - Food and Drug Administration - American federal agency for the control of drugs and food.

this change meant a reduction in the sales volume of national companies (CORDEIRO, 1978).

In Brazil, this process of denationalization of the pharmaceutical industry began in the 1950s. In 1974, there were 529 pharmaceutical companies: 460 national and 69 foreign, of which 10 held 100% of the technical knowledge and monopolized its use. "Although 98% of medicines were industrialized in the country at the time, they were made through simple manipulations, associations between drugs or packaging, etc." This means that, "in reality, 50% of pharmaceuticals, the active ingredients of medicines obtained by extraction, fermentation or synthesis, are imported". In addition, "90% of the drugs on the market are the result of research carried out abroad by the headquarters of large multinational companies" (CORDEIRO, 1978, p. 95).

Products were already promoted by sales reps or laboratory representatives, whose expenses were proportionally similar in domestic and foreign firms. The ratio between salaries and sales commissions in foreign firms was 62.7% and in domestic firms 65.7%; in relation to turnover, it was 12% in both sectors (CORDEIRO, 1978).

The power of capital in the health sector in Brazil is represented by the Medical Industrial Complex - CMI[3] . This is a conglomerate that involves technologies and knowledge, configuring a set of productive activities of which the pharmaceutical industry is a part. Directed by service providers, the consumer market for industrial production is the driving force behind the medical-industrial complex. Therefore, the dynamics of accumulation and innovation in the industry depend on commercial relations (expansion, contraction and the direction of purchases) between suppliers and service providers (GADELHA, 2003).

As a result of its dynamic approach to the health economy, the CMI stands out politically for its participation of private interest groups and the work of organized civil society in drawing up public policies. In the institutional context, it stands out for its relationship with science and technology institutions (GADELHA, 2003).

Reflecting on this process, it is possible to see that, in society's force field, the

[3] The CMI is made up of two large segments: industrial sectors - chemical and biotechnology-based industries and mechanical, electronic and materials-based industries - and service-providing sectors: hospitals, outpatient clinics and diagnostic and treatment services (GADELHA, 2003, p.524).

concept of health and scientific knowledge have the same weight. Considering discourse as a power strategy, to the extent that medical practices have become consumer goods, the medical-industrial complex has been assimilated into the cultural imagination as an indispensable resource for quality medical care. From Foucault's disciplinary perspective, it is a medicalizing device that has become part of the repertoire of popular demands, reinforcing the process of medicalization and sanitarization of society (CAMARGO Jr., 1995).

Since these processes are not always transparent, it is a conflict of interests involving ethical, political and scientific values. The pharmaceutical industry's interference in the production of knowledge, based on the dynamics of consumption, touches on critical points in the epistemic dimension of medicine, because, to the extent that economic interests direct what is or isn't empirical, the credibility of the knowledge-building process is compromised (GREENE, 2007).

Considering that knowledge plays a key role in the medical decision-making process, the replacement of current practices with knowledge presented as new needs to be anchored in legitimate criteria of credibility. However, beyond the false conception that science produces absolute truths, the medical world today is experiencing the contradiction of credibility; a condition that makes doctors vulnerable and colonizes the medical profession (CAMARGO JR., 2007).

Today, enhancing this reality, the scientific, political and social values of the health discourse influence it in such a way that it is enough for scientific knowledge to be disseminated for it to be transformed as early as possible into intervention, both individual and collective. As the biopolitical dimension of medicine, it is this process of sanitarization of life that gives rise to the contemporary doctrine of pharmaceutical prevention. What's more, because it doesn't just involve the doctor, since there is no such thing as a disease, it can reach a large population.

The confluence of marketing and epidemiology has allowed medicines to become crucial in the philosophical definition and promotion of disease. To the extent that disease has become both an epidemiological event and a market event, a peculiar and complex relationship has emerged between medicine and disease, risk and diagnosis, medicine and the market (GREENE, 2007).

The truth is that the concept of the cause of illness can change as a result of changes in medical knowledge. For example, with the emergence of modern medical doctrine, the first anatomopathologists thought it impossible to know the causes of illness. On the other hand, with microbiology came the assumption that the action of microorganisms was the cause of all illnesses. Nowadays, the theoretical perspective of molecular biology revives this illusion through the belief that, with genetic mapping, any disease can be recognized and cured (CAMARGO JR, 1990).

Although in the context of medical knowledge there is no general conceptualization of what illness is, in Foucault's sense, it is possible to describe illnesses as discursive forms, rather than considering them pre-existing. This is a construction of illness, whose generic framework can be identified in three dimensions: explanatory, morphological and semiological (CAMARGO JR., 2003).

The explanatory dimension concerns the pathophysiological process of the disease, the cause of which is established by epidemiology. The morphological dimension is the description of pathognomonic lesions by pathological anatomy. Under the microscope, the lesion is described by its molecular aspect. For this reason, the laboratory paraphernalia of complementary tests is basically aimed at showing lesions. Semiology is the clinical dimension, where the disease is represented by signs and symptoms. In the movement to include the individual case in the nosological grid, the clinic approaches epidemiology, which, by studying diseases in populations, becomes indistinguishable from the clinic (CAMARGO JR., 2003).

Today, the relevance of this issue is due to the fact that the line between normal and pathological has become a numerical alteration. Connected to the statistical probability of developing symptoms in the future, high blood pressure, mild diabetes or high cholesterol are diagnosed as potential risks using laboratory instruments or techniques (GREENE, 2007).

Although the theoretical-conceptual fluidity of medicine means that any epistemological "ruptures" do not necessarily imply ruptures in the clinic, linear causality, as mechanistic thinking, still outlines the scientific imagination of contemporary medicine. However, in the new doctrine of pharmacological prevention, there are no causes of illness, but rather risk factors (CAMARGO JR., 1990).

(2003), the taxonomical production of diseases, based on qualitative and quantitative descriptions, is quite similar when clinics and epidemiology are combined. When establishing causes, it is up to epidemiology to provide clinics with the scientific evidence needed to legitimize them. Insofar as the "objective evidence" of scientificity comes from probabilistic mathematical models, mathematical data tends to be interpreted as a criterion of "truth".

As far as doctors are concerned, it can be said that, either because of their dogmatic reverence for scientific knowledge or because they lack a critical background in experimental methodology, the criteria for assimilating knowledge end up not being a subject for discussion. The consequence of this is that the evidence of empirical experience provided by epidemiology ends up allowing probabilistic data to be interpreted as causal factors (CAMARGO JR., 2003).

This also means that, in the field of biological science, "scientific certainty" is given by the objectivity of signs, even in the absence of symptoms. It is in a composition in which signs are considered more objective and therefore more "scientific" than symptoms that the "scientificity" of the risk doctrine ends up affirming risk factors as the cause of illness (GREENE, 2007).

In the context of contemporary biopolitics, the identification of risk factors has become a "precious" prevention strategy, as it has great potential for providing recommendations. When the doctrine of risk prevention is extended to the entire population, there is a leap in scope never before imagined.

Supported by *guidelines,* this practice has become the mainstay of contemporary medicine. Despite being a shift away from traditional medical fundamentals, the number of ischemia and heart attacks in the United States has declined significantly in recent decades. In addition, hundreds of randomized trials and "placebo-controlled" clinical trials have demonstrated clear benefits in preventing heart disease, ischemia, blindness and kidney failure (GREENE, 2007).

Based on this data, risk-reduction pharmacopoeia should not be seen solely from the perspective of a marketing strategy or a gimmick to increase the turnover of medical practices. Although promotion contributes to the endorsement of drug prescribing, doctors and patients have not simply been bribed by the industry. Public

Health, for example, has advocated the expanded use of these drugs through *lobbying* by respected scientists, eminent clinicians, patient activists and disease communities (GREENE, 2007).

Despite this relativization, it is known that this configuration of power is underpinned by a mechanism that subordinates scientific knowledge to economic interests. In this reality of conflicting interests, we have to consider the Collective Health movement, which, being part of the same force field, tries to direct its interests in the opposite direction to that of the industry. In a dynamic of commitment to public health, it invests in the process of producing and appropriating knowledge according to the health demands of the population.

In addition, reducing costs is essential for public health. As a result of this interest, evidence-based medicine has evolved, as the therapeutic guide *(guideline),* among others, is accompanied by this statement. With the aim of improving the population's quality of health, the *guideline* has been advocated as a strategy for organizing health actions. However, a controversial discussion puts the problem in doubtful terms: is the procedure intended to improve the quality of health or is it intended to increase profits?

The second hypothesis is relevant, insofar as the economic power of pharmaceutical laboratories tends to influence the composition of the *guideline.* In other words, through manipulation strategies, they end up favoring risky pharmacopoeia in the *guideline.* This sets up a strategic conduct in favor of their interests, both in the production of knowledge and in the consumption of their products.

If the function of a *guideline* is to guide practice, and not to limit actions in order to avoid costs, the Ministry of Health should make an effort to issue *guidelines* aimed, at least, at primary care. An investment of this nature could certainly represent a leap in the quality of health actions, as well as resizing the composition of an important field of forces.

# 5 Field Research: The Dynamics of Medical Knowledge Production under the Sponsorship of the Pharmaceutical Industry

## 5.1 Methodology

In order to investigate the dynamics of the production of medical knowledge under the patronage of the pharmaceutical industry, it was considered essential to choose a university hospital as the field of research, since in addition to being a *locus* for the production of academic-scientific knowledge, it is characterized by combining medical care, teaching and research. It is a public institution which, for reasons of confidentiality, will not be identified here.

At this hospital, I conducted semi-structured interviews with four doctors who were professors of medicine and involved in industry-sponsored research. The information gathered was based on three perspectives: the way in which doctors are involved in research, the process of constructing clinical evidence and the doctors' understanding of the contemporary construction of this knowledge.

In accordance with the protocol of the National Research Ethics Commission, the research project was previously submitted to the institution's Research Ethics Committee (CEP), which analyzed and specified any pending issues. After corrections and adjustments, the Committee issued a conclusive opinion approving the project. This process served as a sign of the role that the Ethics Committee is currently playing at the institution. It was implicit that the participation of any medical professional in any research project would depend on the first presentation of a favorable opinion from the CEP.

This requirement seemed to have the function of safeguarding the protectionist nature of doctors, backed by the mantle of ethics. Refining this reflection, it can be said that this is an interpretative analogy of bioethical aspects, which equates the need to protect human beings in biological experiments with the need to avoid inadvertently revealing supposedly inappropriate professional behavior.

Thus, the pending issues pointed out by the Ethics Committee were related to the semi-structuring of questions that left room for the interviewee's understanding. The request to "indicate how the participation of the pharmaceutical industry in the process will be addressed in the interview" was accepted. In order to broaden the "respondent's" view of the investigation into the implicit participation of the industry in the research process, two direct questions were added to the scope of the interview:

1) How does the relationship between the clinical research group and the sponsoring pharmaceutical industry work?

2) What are the dynamics of organizing/selecting articles for publication, in view of the industry as a funder of research?

Also, in response to the Committee's request regarding the question "How do you see the issue of 'conflict of interest'?", it was clarified that this expression has been used to address situations in which there is no convergence between scientific and economic interests. Conflict of interest" has been the focus of attention, especially in terms of its ethical and bioethical aspects. Assimilated as a slogan, the term has come to be cited in editorials and used at medical congresses as a way of giving public credibility to the work presented (GOLDIM, 2006).

Considering that the interests of the industry do not always coincide with those of the doctor or the medical therapist, the question was formulated with the aim of assessing how the doctor deals with the force of the industry's economic power, to the extent that it prioritizes its own interests. I therefore made the question more explicit: "How do you see the issue of 'conflict of interest' between industry and the production of medical knowledge in clinical research processes?"

The fieldwork involved interviews with doctors and professors of medicine involved in clinical research sponsored by the pharmaceutical industry. When the CEP refused to nominate doctors
involved in research with the characteristics mentioned above, the choice of participants was made through the intermediation of medical colleagues who, because they carry out their professional activities at the Institution, are part of the research field, represent trusted people and constitute a reference of loyalty.

These factors favored the approach and selection of the research collaborators, as well as facilitating interaction between the researcher and the interviewees. In order to select the participants from the universe of nominations, professional respectability in the medical field and the academic prominence conferred by their peers were taken into account, in addition to the diversification of medical specialties.

Scheduled directly by telephone with each of those invited to take part in the research, the interviews followed a standardized approach in which the presentation of the Ethics Committee's conclusive opinion was part of the protocol. After preliminary information on the objectives of the research and reiteration of the invitation to take part, adherence was consolidated by signing the Free and Informed Consent Form.

The interviewees were all male, doctors, between 25 and 36 years old, professors at the Faculty of Medicine of the institution, with doctorate degrees in different specialties. Other details about the characteristics of the participants will be kept confidential because, as well as being few in number, they are well-known professionals and therefore easily identifiable. As a privacy strategy, they will be referred to by four fictitious names, namely: Jose, Mauro, Sergio and Luis.

The first three are currently involved in clinical trials funded by the pharmaceutical industry. Luis's inclusion in the research was based on the fact that he was president of a national Society of Specialists, where events, lectures, symposia, congresses, etc. were organized in close partnership with the industry. Also because of his frustrating attempts to take part in multicenter studies. In one of them, ANVISA[4] did not authorize the use of the drug and, in another, the project was rejected by the Institution's Ethics Committee.

The interviews took place in quiet rooms in the respective sectors of the institution where the professionals routinely work. Although busy, with multiple roles (teaching, research and care), all the participants were punctual, welcomed me cordially and allowed the interviews to be recorded.

This was attributed to the relationship of trust established, due to the credibility of the medical colleagues of reference. Likewise, the favorable availability to participate and collaborate in the interviews, which lasted an average of fifty to sixty minutes, can also be credited to this fact.

[4] ANVISA - National Health Surveillance Agency.

The first contact coincided with the moment of the interview, as all the interviewees were strangers. *Rapport* may have been favored by the fact that I was a doctor and part of the same imaginary universe of reference. In addition, my professional experience as a psychiatrist and psychotherapist may have provided a facilitating environment for interactive interviews.

As this is a qualitative method, the meaning and intentionality of these attitudes were valued as part of the research itself, even though we are aware of the theoretical and practical consequences of this approach. Although the value of this interaction is irrefutable, it is known that interpersonal relationships involve aspects that cannot be operationalized in numbers and variables. In Minayo's (1992) proposal, this challenge of the qualitative method can be overcome by using the concept of meaning. According to this author, instead of quantifying the evidence, the meaning of the event must be sought in the intricacies of the experience.

For Minayo (1992), the scientific merit of qualitative research is based on the transferability of sample data to situations with similar characteristics. Since this research cannot be quantified, the qualitative credibility parameters suggested by the author were adhered to. In order to allow peer review to evaluate the results obtained, special care was taken to describe the various stages of the research, taking into account the characteristics, conceptions and procedures of the sample studied.

The transcription of the recordings made during the fieldwork was followed by the search and selection of recurring themes, which were grouped according to their coherence. As Spink (2004) suggests, the choice of themes was a strategic foundation for grasping the perceptions and conceptions embedded in the intertext, whose analysis aims to reconstruct the style of contemporary medical thought. For, in the sense given by Fleck (1979), it is through the process of socialization that the "style of thought" is incorporated into the "collective of thought" - which, for the author, refers to an intellectual community, in other words, a context of interaction between people and the exchange of ideas.

From this perspective, the data was interpreted according to Spink's methodology (2004), in which the production of meanings is studied based on the repertoire of medical discourse. Loaded with meaning, it can be said that the interviewee's opinion is a representation, in other words, it is a voice resulting from *n* voices. In this sense, the object of study in this research - the discourse of the Professor of Medicine funded by the pharmaceutical industry to carry out clinical research - is a protagonist's point of view. Or rather, the *voice,* understood as an enunciation of hegemonic medical languages, is configured within a context in which the protagonist "of the speech" is inserted.

On the other hand, despite this understanding, even with the concept that the enunciation is populated by multiple *voices,* it was impossible to abstract the idea that the enunciation also concerns singular experiences and therefore has an author. Therefore, in order to stimulate the spontaneous reporting of experiences, questions with a broad approach were deliberately drawn up. Although structured questioning was avoided, care was taken to get as close as possible to the object under study.

In discussing the empirical material, the qualitative parameters of credibility were maintained. With reference to the concept of the "meaning" of evidence, the carefully described data was subjectively signified and interpreted. Based on Foucault's conception that the articulation between knowledge and medical power is inseparable, the analysis of the selected themes was based on the articulation between scientific interest and economic power. In the contemporary process of co-production of medical knowledge, the financing role of the pharmaceutical industry was considered in order to study its interaction with the doctor collaborating in the research.

## 5.2 Analysis and Discussion of Results

Considering the role of collaborator in research sponsored by the pharmaceutical industry, the first reading of the testimonies served to verify that, once the objectives of the research had been explained, in the four interviews of the sample under study, the doctors' discourse always had as a reference their interaction with the pharmaceutical industry that was funding them.

Thus, subsequent readings of the material transcribed from the interviews confirmed that all the doctors taking part in this research have a close relationship with the industry, through collaboration in multicenter clinical trials, among other studies, and/or as lecturers in continuing education programs to promote the products.

Because of their familiarity with this dynamic, the doctors interviewed show that they know how this interaction works and the criticisms involved. Insofar as they live with the conflict of interests inherent in the process, their discourses seek coherence with ethical, political and scientific principles.

It's worth noting that one doctor was accurately indicated by other professors, with the information that she was carrying out clinical research sponsored by a pharmaceutical laboratory. This was confirmed by telephone and the interview was scheduled. After a delay of an hour and a half, the doctor arrived at her consulting room and apologized for having to see the representatives of the laboratories before the interview, whom she usually met at that time. After explaining the research, the doctor signed the Free and Informed Consent Form, and then kindly provided the information that she was not carrying out any research sponsored by the pharmaceutical industry. Considering the voluntary nature of the invitation, an analysis of this fact points to a possible refusal to take part in the research.

(2007), it is known that an important part of research activities, as well as the production and distribution of biomedical knowledge, is largely under the control of private commercial interests. Therefore, in their speeches, the doctors interviewed did not neglect the possibility of expressing their opinions on the importance of the pharmaceutical industry's participation in research processes.

Considering the university environment as a space for building knowledge, they justify taking part in clinical research. On the other hand, they regret the university's failure to take advantage of the investment opportunity offered by the pharmaceutical industry.

> "[...] when we understand that research is important [...] I've been working here with this smaller part, which is research linked to the pharmaceutical industry" (Jose).
>
> "[...] It's very complex to build this in the university environment, which

doesn't have an organized structure for it. [...] It's really a loss of opportunity" (Jose).

"Although the government has invested three and a half million reais here to build a clinical research unit, to [...], with these contracts with the pharmaceutical industry, guarantee independence [...] the institution doesn't respond as it should" (Jose).

"One of the important points is that, in order to build a clinical trial, there has to be an environment of professionalization, of laboratory results, of people, of the structure as a whole" (Jose).

"Without this, you can't develop clinical research that can receive an FDA audit, be approved, and receive constant monitoring and be approved" (Jose).

"It's something that you can lose the opportunity to have new drugs if you lose that investment" (Jose).

With evident assimilation of the industry's discourse on the "risks" inherent in pharmaceutical research, the interviewees recognize the expansion of the area of drug research, highlighting the clinical benefits brought about by technological innovation. On the other hand, the increase in health care costs is critically attributed to the pharmaceutical industry.

"Because of the costs of multicenter research [...] pharmaceutical research *is* a risky investment, as many studies give negative or neutral results" (Jose).

"Laboratories are researching new weapons, new medicines" (Luis).

"Currently, I'm doing more clinical research, [...] work related to epidemiology" (Mauro).

"We're getting ready to take on some studies for the pharmaceutical industry, to study some new drugs in various areas" (Mauro).

"The construction of (medical) knowledge has evolved more in the last five years than in the last fifty years. There has been a profound technological therapeutic evolution" (Jose).

"Thanks to preventive measures and technological innovation [...] people's survival and quality of life has changed" (Jose).

"But, of course, many advances today are translated into clinical benefits; which are not just blood pressure control, in other words, the individual having fewer heart attacks, fewer strokes, fewer sequelae, less kidney failure, and somehow reducing costs" (Jose).

"The criticism of the pharmaceutical industry is precisely because these advances have led to a huge increase in the cost of medical care" (Jose).

However, when they highlight the commercial interest of the industry, they confirm Angell's (2007) argument that most laboratories channel their investments into advertising and marketing, rather than investing in innovation. They even favor the reproduction of drugs already consolidated on the market as a profit strategy.

> "It is now a high-cost industry, which has also channeled part of its profits and internal costs [...] into advertising and marketing, which 'unbalances' this relationship" (Jose).
> "There are laboratories [...] interested in innovation. There are about ten. But there are many more laboratories copying medicines than innovating" (Jose).

> "It's a business; if they invest, it's because they earn. [...] the biggest industries are pharmaceuticals. [...] and they make money from us doctors" (Mauro).
> "[...] there has been a great technological advance driven by a company or group of companies whose core is profit (Тсзё).
> "And there's the commercial interest" (Luis).
> "[...] the ones who have the money today to subsidize research are the laboratories. It matters a lot to them [the laboratories]" (Mauro).

The majority of multicenter studies are phase IV studies, i.e. they involve drugs that have already been approved and are now being tested for a different indication. This is the case with anticonvulsants, which are now being used as mood stabilizers. This is a marketing strategy by the pharmaceutical industry, with the aim of expanding the drug's range of action and thus boosting profits.

> "These are drugs that are already practically instituted in other countries. So it's to see if the efficacy rate is the same in Brazil" (Luis).
> "Most of the time, these studies are very important, because the laboratory, in order to release the drug with another indication (...) has to come here and test it on the Brazilian population [...]" (Mauro).
> "[...] they appear as anticonvulsants, then they see that they also serve as mood stabilizers and so they are applied to migraine, with the same response" (Luis).
> "So what happens? We usually catch this patient in stage IV" (Luis).

As far as remuneration is concerned, some doctors who collaborate in research, while considering it pertinent, try to convey the idea of a greater interest for the sake of science. But in reality, the contracts for this work establish payment per patient recruited, or for a previously stipulated monthly amount.

"In financial terms, the pay is very unattractive. It's a lot of work and they pay very little. Participating in research has to be for the scientific aspect, not for what you earn" (Crgio).
"[...] as lead investigator, I earn around 600 reais a month. The investigators get 300 reais a month" (Crgio).
"[...] they pay us per patient we include. I include, in this case, 15 patients" (Mauro).

"It would be paid research. Around 120 reais per patient (taken), plus the money for the patient's ticket" (Luis).
"[...] it has a sharing policy: part of the money goes to the university and the other part belongs to the researcher and the people who take part in the research" (Тсзё).
"In terms of financing, either they pay per patient you include or they already set an **x** amount for you to receive at that time. But generally, it's per patient you include" (Mauro).
"In this research [specialized support reference], I don't even receive anything, but I could be receiving it, because for each consultation [...], they would pay around forty-something reais, based on the AMB table" (Mauro).

Some of the doctors interviewed clearly explained the nature of the collaboration sought by the drug industry. In some cases, the invitation to participate in clinical trials under their sponsorship is restricted to the role of patient recruiter. As well as giving greater credibility to studies, university hospitals offer a greater possibility of attracting and selecting patients, either because of the quantity of human material or because of the greater concentration of pathological diversity. In this case, doctors, who are university professors, are the technicians whose profile best combines the attributes capable of meeting this demand, which, incidentally, is very well exploited by the pharmaceutical industry.

"What we use is human resources. We have too many patients, and they [the laboratories] have too few" (Luis).
"This has to be done within the university centers, because it's something that has to go through the Ethics Committee" (Mauro).
"I'm taking part in a study with patients who are basically hard to find, but we managed to select some patients" (Mauro).
"The protocol is done by the laboratory itself. I'm simply involved [...] executing the protocol, that's all. [...] I'm just someone hired to recruit patients" (S'rgio).
"[...] they had to expand this research, because they couldn't find enough patients to study the product better and make the link. So they had to expand the centers. They ended up here in Brazil" (Mauro).

Regarding the selection of participants in clinical trials, the mechanisms used by the pharmaceutical industry are explained as follows:

> "[...] my contact with the laboratory staff was at the time of selection. An evaluator and a monitor came to find out about my training, curriculum and previous research experience" (Mauro).
> "In general, they select you on the computer [...] based on your CV. If they're interested in patients with 'a certain disease'; see who publishes it [...] and they'll find you" (Sergio).
> "I received an e-mail that read: 'I am writing to you on behalf of so-and-so, who represents the pharmaceutical industry, with the aim of locating world opinion leaders regarding the clinical management of this disease'" (Sergio).
> "I mean, [...] he goes online and, as he clearly says, 'we did some bibliographical research and noticed that you have recently published in this area'. And they ask if I have *'interesting personal participation in clinical treatment'"* (Sergio).
> "[...] in general, asking me to point out 6 to 8 opinion formers, or experts in the area [under study], in Brazil and in the world, that they can contact" (Sergio).

In multi-centre projects funded by the pharmaceutical industry, there are a series of requirements in the choice of institution, research participants and team organization, the dynamics of which are defined by the interviewees as complex, laborious and careful. For some, this has a particular meaning of rigor and seriousness on the part of the industry.

> "It's a lot of work, because they're very strict with the forms. It's a lot of 'little forms'. We send it [...], they send it back" (Mauro).
> "[...] when I assign someone, I have to send all the data to the laboratory. It's a lot of work, they're very strict and demanding. This spreadsheet here, for example, shows the names of the people involved, the job each person does and how much they earn per month" (Sergio).
> "[This research] went through a very strict evaluation. I was having difficulty [...] but, over time, I managed to be chosen" (Mauro).
> "So it's a very serious study, very serious indeed. So much so that there was a survey that we didn't take part in, [...] it wasn't within the specifications" (Mauro).
> "They are often very strict in their criteria, because these are studies that are going to be published in high-impact international journals; and the journals are very rigorous in their analysis" (Mauro).
> "Research into [this drug] has been going on for almost two years. It includes Brazil. We were one of the centers chosen, there's one in Sao Paulo and another, I think, in Minas" (Mauro).
> "They were finding it difficult to include, because they are very strict when it comes to entry, when choosing these centers" (Mauro).

It is an organizational structure made up of a chain of hierarchical roles, with varying degrees of responsibility. There is a team from the pharmaceutical industry itself that links up with third-party firms, making up a complex chain of coordinators, monitors and local, national and international researchers/collaborators.

> "[...] every study has a local principal investigator - *PI (Principal Investigator)"* (Sergio).
> "I'm the PI of this study. So I select [...] a study coordinator, who will be my right-hand man in the administrative management of the project; [...] I choose the medical team, the investigators and, eventually, some medical support" (Sergio).
> "I had the opportunity to be the coordinator of a local research project and the national coordinator of a clinical trial, as part of a network of collaborators" (Jose).
> "The (principal) investigators are not necessarily doctors from the pharmaceutical industry, but university professors from America and Europe, who have obtained support from the industry to carry out the research or have been asked by the industry to take part in a clinical trial to validate a therapeutic hypothesis" (Jose).
> "It's not really the laboratory staff who come. They hire a company, which works with a specific monitor, who comes from time to time" (Mauro).

In practice, this organizational composition constitutes strategic distancing, both between the members of the various arms of the research and between the multiple centers where the research has been implemented. This dynamic can be translated as an intentional and perverse lack of communication between the central international research coordinator and the local principal investigator of each clinical trial.

Strategically designed, the programmatic movement, with the air of strict monitoring of scientific criteria, is nothing more than a production plant for clinical evidence, whose setting in itself needs to convey credibility and scientific legitimacy to the knowledge produced.

> "There is the figure of the monitor, responsible for the research, who monitors the progress of the research during each period, to verify the rigidity of the criteria they have established" (Mauro).
> "No one has access. All contacts are made through me or the study coordinator. Even so, the study coordinator, most of the time, goes through me" (Sergio).
> "At the moment, I don't have any more contact. It's the project coordinator

> who receives the visits" (Mauro).
> "When you have a study like this with different areas at work, you're kind of isolated in the research. We get in touch with each other, we talk, but it's more on paper. There's not much direct contact" (Mauro).
> "Sometimes there's a meeting with everyone, because there are several people from different areas. There's a specialized part for each piece of research" (Mauro).

When referring to the drafting of multicenter study protocols, doctors clearly verbalize the mechanisms by which the sponsoring industry team excludes them from the process.

> "It usually happens like this: they call you to a meeting in the preliminary phase, they discuss where the project is at" (Sergio).
> "When you're a principal investigator on a project like this, you're taking part in a discussion on a protocol that has already been discussed and approved" (Jose).
> "The protocol is drawn up by the laboratory's own staff. I wasn't involved in designing the protocol." (Sergio).
> "The criteria are set by them. They defend them. The protocol is all theirs, and they are extremely difficult criteria. We have to send the tests to them. The laboratories are appointed by them" (Mauro).

In this context, although it is possible to see in one of the interviewees the illusion of active participation in decisions, in reality, invitations to meetings, with promises of discussion, seem to be no more than a formality to legitimize the process.

> "In this phase, [...] there is a lot of opportunity to add more items to the protocol. The discussion is broader [...], a set of questions is raised and discussed with the national coordinators." (Jose)
> "[...] if there is some kind of ethical problem, you are free either not to accept the project or to send a suggestion to the national coordinator so that he can contact the central investigators of the work" (Josd).
> "It's a superficial view to think that the pharmaceutical industry shoves whatever protocol it wants down our throats. In reality, this has existed for a long time. The focus of research was on the efficacy aspect" (Josd).
> "[...] a final version [of the project], approved by international researchers [...] and then sent to the different centers" (Jose).

In one of the multicenter studies developed by one of the collaborators, the research protocol was presented as closed. As the invitation to participate meant joining an ongoing clinical trial, with a large number of patients already recruited, the possibility of any changes to the protocol was practically nil. However, the announced meeting to discuss the protocol did take place.

> "They called me to the meeting. I know the questions and I took part in the discussion, in the changes to the protocol." (Sdrgio).
> "[...] they allow small changes to the protocol; if you give them a relevant opinion, they may even change something, but most of the time they don't" (Sdrgio).
> "In this work, for example, the work was already underway with more than 1400 patients recruited" (Sdrgio).
> "It was my first experience of this kind of multicenter, international work, in the United States, in Europe, all over the world" (Sergio).
> "I'm just a person hired to recruit [patients]. I simply take part [...] by executing the protocol, that's all" (Sdrgio).

From this perspective, it is possible to grasp, at the same time, the ethical and scientific dimensions of a study involving a serious illness, the drug being evaluated is aimed at treating a complication of the disease, i.e. a worsening of the condition. Patients are routinely monitored by the researchers in accordance with the study protocol, taking notes, recording and reporting.

> "The question that this research seeks to answer is: if we treat anemia in diabetic patients who have chronic renal failure, even in the pre-dialysis phase, does this reduce cardiovascular mortality?" (Crgio).
> "This study seeks to use a drug that interferes with the synthesis of red blood cells. If patients with controlled hematocrit [...] had lower cardiovascular mortality" (Crgio).
> "As principal investigator, I don't see that patient. [...] Two sub-researchers [...] see the patients on a regular basis, or whenever the patient deems it necessary" (Crgio).
> "If the patient is admitted to a hospital with a health insurance, outside of here, we have an obligation to go there and find out what happened, [...] see what complications the patient had" (Crgio).
> "We behave as if we are responsible for all the patient's information, even if they happen to have a health plan and are admitted to another hospital. We have to go there" (Crgio).

Although these patients, recruited and included in this double-blind clinical trial, require permanent clinical and laboratory monitoring, the doctors involved in the investigation, as well as not having access to the results of the laboratory tests, do not know whether they are administering placebo or active substance to the patients under their medical care.

> "So what do we do? It's a double-blind study. We don't really know what we're administering. All the medication comes in the mail, to be administered in identical syringes" (Crgio).
> "I don't have access to the hemoglobin values [of the tests] that the lab does. [...] I don't have access, but he tells me the critical point." * / ',5rgio)
>
> "Now, if a patient becomes ill at any time and goes to the emergency room, any doctor can order a hematocrit and find out what their hemoglobin level is. I mean, this question doesn't involve ... [greater risk? [greater risk?]" (Crgio).

According to the principal investigator, as part of the protocol, there is a rescue point, the need for which is indicated by the hematocrit[5] and the hemoglobin level[6] , both of which are checked in the blood test. When the hemoglobin level is equal to or less than 9 (nine), because it involves a risk to the patient, it is characterized as an emergency. At this critical point, the industry tells the investigating doctor that the patient needs to be treated urgently. In this circumstance, it is perhaps redundant to point out that this rescue point is demanded by patients who are "blindly" using placebo.

Considering that the "limit" of risk is in the hands of the industry, and not under the control of the attending physician, it is worth mentioning Sayd's (2006) considerations on the physician's departure from traditional medical values. In addressing the incorporation of technological advances into medical practice, the author recognizes a shift in the doctor-patient relationship, such as loss of autonomy and loss of the monopoly of care over the patient.

---

[5] The hematocrit is an index, measured in the blood test, calculated as a percentage, defined by the volume of all the red blood cells in a sample over the total volume of this sample. Normal reference values in adults range from 40 - 50% in men and 36 - 45% in women. In chronic renal failure, a hematocrit between 33% and 36% is considered normal.

[6] Hemoglobin (often abbreviated as Hb) is the pigment that gives red blood cells their color. It is a metalloprotein that contains iron and has the function of transporting oxygen to the tissues. In chronic renal failure, the level considered normal ranges from 11g/dl to 12g/dl.

> "[...] there is a rescue point, that is, if, by chance, the patient's hematocrit falls below 9, which is considered a risk for the person being treated in the blind spot, the Central Laboratory says: Look, you have a patient at the critical point, with a hematocrit of 9 or less, you need to treat this patient" (Sergio)[7] .
> "He [the laboratory] warns us because, as it's a placebo-controlled study, there's a risk that people who aren't taking the drug will become critically anemic. But there is the concern of a limit, which is detected by the laboratory" (Sergio).

The discussion about the bioethical dimension of the use of placebos was also supported by another doctor interviewed. Because it involved the use of placebos, his research project was rejected by the institution's Ethics Committee.

> "Some time ago, we tried to develop a study. But it involved the placebo group" (Luis).
> "It's just that the Ethics Committee here hasn't authorized the use of placebo. [...] I don't know why, but they think it will prolong the pain" (Luis).

And, in favor of the use of placebo, he takes as argumentative reinforcement the reference of the International Society of his Specialty which, according to the report, not only approves the use of placebos in clinical trials, but also conditions the work to this protocol.

> "It's interesting to have the placebo group, because if you consider that 30% of placebos work [on pain], that is, if you give the placebo to a population of 100 patients with pain, around 30% of the individuals will respond" (Luis).
> "So we're obliged to give a placebo. This is stated in the world literature; without it, the International Society won't accept it as work" (Luis).
> "We came up with a scheme of giving the drug, [...] knowing who was using the active substance and who was using the placebo" (Luis).
> "We used to stipulate: if you're in pain for up to two hours after taking the medication, you can use one of the drugs you're used to, to abort the crisis. But they wouldn't let us" (Luis).
> "Now, those patients [...] who have the resource to meet the researcher whenever they want, have a hospital of this size to attend to them, [...] and

7 In the interview recording, the reference to the hematocrit leaves no doubt. However, a hematocrit of 9 is so absurdly low that it is impossible to rule out the possibility of a mistake. It is possible that the interviewee said hematocrit when he was actually referring to the hemoglobin value. This in no way changes the logical line of analysis regarding the risks that the patient is being subjected to in the investigation.

> even so, [the research project] is not accepted?" (Luis).

He says that this has often been the case in his attempts to develop clinical studies. He criticizes the actions of the Ethics Committee, considering them to be an impediment to the development of drug research, and attributes to the committee a lack of scientific vision.

> "I haven't yet had the chance to test a new medication. I'd like to" (Luis).
> "[...] I've had [difficulties with the Ethics Committee] several times. We even lost an excellent position; an international multicenter study with a type of medicine. They wouldn't let us" (Luis).
> "It was the Jansen laboratory. It was [...] Denmark, [...] the United States doing it at the same time. And Brazil was privileged [in the choice], [...] but they wouldn't let us. It died. It stopped there. Then Peru and Bolivia did it" (Luis).

> "[...] with one of the laboratories, we tried to do the research and Anvisa banned it [...] in the United States, there started to be side effects in the research there, so they didn't allow it to be tested here" (Luis).
> "If [...] the Ethics Committees had a more uniform concept [...] it would make this drug research much easier" (Luis).
> "I see this as a complete lack of scientific vision" (Luis).
> "[there is] a need to change the Committee's vision, without which they will kill part of the research, especially in the development of medicines" (Luis).

Maintaining a fervent argument about the use of placebo in drug trials, the interviewee does not consider any bioethical commitment in his proposal, and even questions traditional ethical references in medical practice. He relativizes and minimizes the suffering of the "poor" who seek care at the university hospital, attributing to them the possibility of tolerating pain, which is indefensible according to the most basic human principles.

> "Research *is* natural. You do it with volunteers, you do it socially and, why not, this return to the use of medicines, the observation of a product in an attempt to improve it" (Luis).
> "Of course there are precepts, all the criteria to protect the individual. You're not going to use a medicine that has already been researched, [...] and not approved" (Luis).
> "Because poor people sometimes come to the emergency room after being in

pain for six hours. Why can't he spend two [hours] without pain relief?" (Luis).
"In theory, because if he [the patient] isn't using the placebo, he might only be [in pain] for half an hour. So [...] he has a chance [of getting relief from the pain]" (Luis).
"I think that this vision, for the university environment, [...] leaves a lot to be desired" (Luis).
"Because [...] there will be an informed consent form, [...] medical support for any resource, 24 hours a day, the researcher's phone, including a cell phone. So I didn't see any difficulty" (Luis).

One of the multicenter research projects, in which three of the doctors interviewed take part, involves different specialties studying the same substance, sponsored by the same pharmaceutical industry. Insofar as, from a bioethical point of view, the use of placebo poses a risk to the patient, the argumentative threshold of the discussion is questionable to say the least.

Based on the search for clinical benefits for chronic kidney disease patients (the subject of the study), this is a drug whose application relativizes, on the one hand, a warning from the FDA *(Food and Drug Administration)* regarding the cardiovascular risk in the evolutionary process of this pathology, and, on the other, the existence of studies that indicate an improvement in the clinical condition of these patients. The reports below provide support for verifying possible contradictions in the approach of an investigation that is already underway.

"[...] it is a drug that has received a warning from the FDA regarding cardiovascular risk when correcting anemia, especially in chronic kidney disease patients" (Cë).
"People [in laboratories] are worried about those with chronic renal failure in the pre-dialysis phase, because those who go on dialysis are survivors. The vast majority die of cardiovascular complications" (Sc'rgio).
"I'm carrying out research into the use of a drug that is currently being discussed by the Research Ethics Committee."
"And the *American Generic* - AMGEN laboratory, [...] which still doesn't have any medicines in Brazil" (Crgio).
"This research [...] is very important, because [...] patients who develop chronic renal failure have anemia, and we have difficulty treating them" (Tc3ë).
"[...] there are some studies that show that improving anemia improves the clinical condition of these patients" (Tc3ë).

As for the results of the research, full access to them is the exclusive preserve of the central coordinators, members of the industry team. In the name of secrecy, of supposed rigor in the conduct of clinical trials, doctors have no access to partial research data, such as drug dosages or laboratory test results. This withholding of essential data related to the use of placebo prevents the investigating doctor from even knowing which patient is taking a placebo or an active substance.

To the same extent that it seeks impartiality and objectivity of results, this makes it impossible to subjectively analyze clinical responses - a dimension, it must be said, that is essential in the drug correlation of subjective pathological mechanisms.

According to the testimonies, the results are presented in the form of summaries, after being evaluated and selected by staff assigned to this task.

> "When it's a blind study, we don't know anything. We don't know if the patient is using the substance or not" (Mauro).
> "The database of these works is not public, it is under the tutelage of the *'sponsors'* of the pharmaceutical industry and central researchers" (Tc3ë).
> "Regional collaborators can have access [...], as long as they contact these principal investigators of the work" (Tc3ë).
> "They give feedback on specific issues" (Tc3ë).
> "The results are presented after [...] they have been summarized" (Tc3ë).

As explained in the speeches, there are contracts in which participating in the publication of results is part of the agreement; but in others, the researcher is made to sign a document, giving up their participation. In this way, the publication of articles containing the results of research is under the absolute power of the interests of the pharmaceutical industry.

> "[...] one of the agreements [...] is to publish the results that have been found" (Luis).
> "[...] I'm not a co-author of the work when it's published. Nothing. We sign a document agreeing that this will be the case" (Sc'rgio).
> "[...] there is a very big 'forgiveness' of the laboratory. Obviously they are important; nowadays, you can't do research without a laboratory, you can't do a congress without a laboratory, you can't publish a journal without a laboratory" (Mauro).
> "Today, without advertising, you can't maintain a medical magazine. So that's the reality. The laboratory plays an important role in this respect. Even because they invest a lot, a lot in research, a lot, a lot of money" (Mauro).

As Angell (2007) points out, *ghost-writers* hired by the pharmaceutical industry are "*ghost* scientists" who assume authorship of a study in which they did not participate. To the extent that this in itself means manipulation by the original writers of the research, it raises ethical questions about the interests involved in concealing the results.

> "They're the ones who evaluate what's going to be published. They take the data from these patients, analyze it within the framework of a strict evaluation and then a publication will come out. Then the name of us and all the centers that took part in the study will be included" (Mauro).
> "I don't publish anything. It's already in the contract. I'm just a patient recruiter" (Sergio).
> "But in practice, we don't write the article; we help provide the data, but we don't write it. Someone else writes it" (Mauro).
> "If you take part, you publish; you get the seal of publication. You can publish fragments of your work, but you have to go through a bureaucracy. You submit your hypothesis to a central committee. The principal investigators from the pharmaceutical industry analyze it. With the agreement of the General Coordinator of the study, if it's accepted, you publish it with the group of researchers." (Jose).
> "The control is in the sense of the unfolding of the research. The *draft of* the clinical research already defines the questions from which it is not possible to distance oneself" (Josë).
> "There are other studies, like the one that was done recently, which has a guy who is responsible for sitting down and doing everything, writing and publishing the article" (Mauro).

In addressing the power of the pharmaceutical industry in the production of medical knowledge, Angell (2007) highlights the industry's influence on medical research, saying that "the clear aim was to bias the data to ensure that their drugs performed well" (p. 16).

In this sense, the dissemination of new drugs and their clinical indications has become a strategy for directly interfering in the possibility of changing prescriptive practices. This constitutes an investment which, supported by scientific discourse, legitimizes clinical research and gives disguised credibility to commercial interests.

This aspect is raised by one of the interviewees, who, while admitting the existence of the problem, puts the marketing strategies into perspective between "inappropriate consumerism and the incorporation of criticism of the drug", to say that today this issue is "identified as a minor problem". And, as shown in fragments of his speech, he explains what he considers to be "the bigger problem"

> "[...] in relation to prescribing, the role of the pharmaceutical industry often distorting results and magnifying the results of benefits, giving little emphasis to safety, in reality, this today is identified as a minor problem" (Jose).
> "[...] the industry has a role of spending more resources on publicizing to the population [...] than on publicizing to doctors. It creates [...] a certain inappropriate consumerism or incorporation of criticism of the medicine" (Jose). "The biggest problem is: are patients taking what they should be taking? Are patients taking the drugs that actually reduce morbidity and mortality? Are their clinical indicators adequate?" (Jose)

This approach outlines the thinking style of the doctors interviewed, in the sense given by Fleck (1979): a medical practice based on a totalizing intellectual disposition, focused on the need to find the biological mechanism of the disease. In the midst of the forces of economic power, this contradiction takes on greater dimension to the exact extent that the production of medical knowledge, dominated by biology, makes the critical capacity of doctors vulnerable. For, as Canguilhem (2006) points out, despite the efforts to rationalize science, the essence of medicine remains clinical and therapeutic.

> "[The patient's] blood pressure is under control, his cholesterol is under control, he's stopped smoking, he's been advised to stop smoking, he's doing physical activity, his HDL is under control, his waistline is adequate? That's what matters in medical practice" (Jose).
> "What is quality? Clinical outcomes and patient safety. Patient safety is what? Proper prescribing, patient orientation, drug compatibility, drug adherence, proper pharmacovigilance system" (Jose).
> "So, the use of a [medicine] [...] that improves the patient's quality of life [...] has great validity" (Mauro).

On the other hand, the impregnation of the pharmaceutical perspective captured here clearly reflects the influence of industry interests on medical thinking. This is a dynamic through which clinical reasoning is being dimensioned from the perspective of clinical pharmacology, and clinical medicine, along the lines of pharmacological doctrine, is being re-dimensioned as pharmaceutical care. The arguments of one of the interviewees bear witness to this line of analysis.

> "[...] our demands today are great in relation to the need to have new ways of treating patients and also to understand the side effects of medicines" (Jose).
> "[...] prescribing [...] often with 20 items. [...] we have to question aspects [...] of the fragmentation of medical knowledge" (Josd).
> "[...] There is a great need for knowledge of clinical pharmacology, for a multidisciplinary view in the therapeutic approach to diseases" (Josd).
> "With the end of therapeutics courses at universities, there is a very large *gap* between knowledge [...] about therapeutics and the critical analysis of therapeutics [...]" (Josd).
> "How can we [...] promote quality pharmaceutical care if we don't have a specific pharmacology and pharmacists interacting?" (Josd).
> "[...] a policy of quality in pharmaceutical care, where the training of pharmacists and multidisciplinary integration are critical when it comes to treating the patient" (Jose).

Furthermore, extrapolating the effective therapeutic action of drugs to treat diseases, the defense of the pharmaceutical doctrine is based on "treating" the potential risk of becoming ill - whether through the control of clinical indicators considered healthy or laboratory data, such as the use of statins to maintain lipid levels within the new standards of normality. This style of thinking is supported by a well-structured discourse:

> "In my opinion, the focus [of medicine] is changing a lot" (Mauro). "[...] the criteria for diabetes are much stricter in relation to altered glucose tolerance" (Mauro).
> "We start treating patients before they become diabetic. They don't have a disease; they just have an alteration, an intolerance to glucose; that would be pre-diabetic. You can prevent the progression of diabetes" (Mauro).
> "There are already industry studies on diabetes prevention [...] showing fantastic results. There's an American government study; [...] an excellent Finnish study" (Mauro).
> "And there's another important thing about cholesterol. Type II diabetics are known to have a very high cardiovascular risk. So you should use a statin as a treatment, even if he hasn't had a heart attack and has never had any damage. Just because he's diabetic" (Mauro).

In this way, the "production of disease" has become an important commercial strategy for the pharmaceutical industry. It involves, at the same time, the pathologization of physiological conditions and the expansion of the concept of disease to mild or pre-symptomatic forms. In this mechanism, "high cholesterol" and pre-diabetic states, which were previously risk factors, have been elevated to the category of disease, based on their risk potential. If diagnosed by laboratory tests, it indicates the need for medication (MOYNIHAN and HENRY, 2006).

A relevant example of this is statins. Initially presented as cholesterol reducers, this group of substances is now being investigated as to their potential action in reducing atheromatous plaques. Although there is recognition of the pressure from the pharmaceutical industry to prescribe statins, a logic of prevention predominates in contemporary medical thinking.

> "Nowadays, prevention is what I think you have to do. It's much better to treat a person before they have the disease, rather than with the disease already established" (Mauro).
> "There is a "forgiveness" of the bar in relation to statins. But in practice, if you really evaluate it, the studies show that mortality is linked to high LDL. And when you reduce LDL, you reduce mortality. It really does!" (Mauro).
> "Today, we're working on something else, which is the reduction of atheromatous plaque with the use of statins" (Mauro).
> "There have already been two studies on statins, and a study is coming out now showing that the problem isn't the drug, it's not rosuvastatin Crestor®, it's the statin itself" (Mauro).
> "If you reduce cholesterol, LDL cholesterol by 50%, you can even reduce plaques. This is independent of the type of statin; any of them" (Mauro).
> "[...] this shows that there is a plate effect. Now, [...] there is a lot of manipulation" (Mauro).

In line with the strategy of producing diseases based on the concept of risk potential, the pharmaceutical industry is currently investing in defining subclinical hypothyroidism in order to defend the hormone dosage threshold at which patients should be treated. According to one of the interviewees, it is called subclinical hypothyroidism when the level of TSH increase does not yet justify prescribing medication. In the reports below, we can see how the industry is going about this process, in order to configure hypothyroid disease.

> "Subclinical hypothyroidism is when you have an elevation in TSH, but it's not so high that you need to treat the patient" (Mauro).
> "The American Thyroid Society and other very serious societies have

defined the following: that you only have to treat the individual who has a TSH higher than 10. And, below 10, if they have some clinical condition, dyslipidemia, a very large goiter, very high antibodies [...], there are the crystals" (Mauro).

"The laboratory wants to show that this person who has a slightly increased TSH already has a risk. [...] There's a lot of discussion!" (Mauro) "For the laboratory, TSH goes up to four and a bit. So they want to show that a patient, for example, with a TSH of 6 (six), normal, is at risk. So they take a guy with a TSH of 3 and a normal T4 and call it subclinical hypothyroidism" (Mauro).

"And [the laboratory] produces a disease. And there are many cases in which we know that a slightly increased TSH can be normal in that person" (Mauro).

"There is a very interesting study from Colorado that showed that there is a large percentage of the population that has a higher TSH level."

"But there are some doctors who join in the dance" (Mauro).

It is in this sense that the dissemination of the results of clinical trials has the main objective of interfering in the prescriptive practices of doctors, in order to produce changes that enhance the use of medicines. The industry's discourse, that it is necessary to change prescriptive habits, was assimilated in such a way by one of the interviewees, that the difficulties of change appear in the intertext of his discourse, represented by barriers (social, cultural and economic) to be faced and modified. And it seems that in promoting their medicines, the pharmaceutical industry's marketing strategies are aimed at tackling "these barriers".

"Why is it that a certain drug, which is effective in the clinical trial, isn't reaching the top, i.e. isn't being prescribed by the doctor? What are the social, cultural and economic barriers to prescribing habits? Why doesn't it reach the top?" (Тсзё).

Then, supported by the results of research, the strategies for presenting new therapeutic proposals take place in various ways: in a big way, at medical congresses, in lectures given under the patronage of the industry, by way of updating or continuing education; or in doctors' surgeries, through representatives of the pharmaceutical industry.

"[...] new drugs are publicized at medical congresses and/or local meetings with opinion leaders, or access to medical literature that reaches the doctor" (Jose).

> "[...] the glamor of congresses in five-star hotels, which create the conditions for an exaggerated view of the results over the impact of the benefits" (Jose).
> "Knowledge comes through lectures, congresses, specialization courses. The doctor in the clinic generally doesn't have much access to journals, he doesn't read much, he doesn't follow closely."
> This knowledge reaches the doctor at the end of the line basically through these actions carried out by the laboratories" (Jose).

As far as congresses are concerned, it can be said that they are a major undertaking, the dynamics of which revolve around the pharmaceutical industry. The vast majority of them are financed by the industries that buy or rent *stands* from the organizing societies. The costs inherent in scientific events are covered by negotiating space for the pharmaceutical trade fair, which is publicized through the distribution of giveaways, *folders,* articles, magazines, books and all sorts of advertising and marketing material.

> "[...] in general practice, [...] 90% of Congresses are sponsored by laboratories" (Luis).
> "It's with the rental of those stands that the boards [of the societies] are going to provide those who are going to pass on the experiences with the payment of tickets, accommodation, etc." (Luis).
> "Congress revolves around this industry, which is there as a showcase. Now it's a business. You're in Rua da Alfandega, you go into the store, and the guy sells you a suitable product. The product is bound to do that" (Luis).
> "[...] they rent stands, they go and sell their fish there" (Luis).
> "[...] doctors will come with an interest in learning, but these doctors will also circulate in the 'market', you know? And there's interest if there's something new, if there are new things, why not?" (Luis).

In addition to funding congresses, the pharmaceutical industry provides funds to "bankroll" doctors who occupy prominent positions in medical specialty societies or to reward doctors who prescribe their products by "sending" them to congresses of their interest, paying for registration, airfare and accommodation.

The first case concerns policies of interest to the industry, related to medical institutions and positions of power. Here, the discourse rules out the possibility of direct interference in prescriptive practices.

> "[...] universities, class societies and medical associations [...] today live dependent on the support of the pharmaceutical industry" (Josd).
> "I'm always invited. Not just by the Society [...], the Brazilian Academy of [specialty] itself invites me to Congress every two years. Of course, this

> funding [...] is via the laboratory" (Luis).
> "Now, I don't see the doctor's participation as deleterious, because he's being paid to go to a congress, with his stay paid for, etc." (Luis).
> "Will this interfere with the behavior of doctors? I've never seen it myself. Not even in theory for me. I've never changed my prescription because... [the laboratory wants it]" (Luis).
> "The Society invited me, through the laboratory; so, with that, I'm going to pass on the medicine from the laboratory? I can't believe it!" (Luis).

In the second case, the negotiation is part of a set of marketing strategies aimed at increasing drug consumption. The proposal may come from the doctor or the industry representative, but what is always at stake is the number of prescriptions for a given product, stipulated by the sales representative.

However, in the intertext of one of the speeches, the insinuation of prescribing drugs without indications is put in terms of the industry improperly selecting who it will give the bonus to. Insofar as what is at stake in the negotiation arena is the quantity of drugs prescribed, this indicates a perversion in the analysis of the problem, since this opening, as a marketing strategy, is given by the industry itself.

> "There is one thing today, which has to do with what laboratories are beginning to see that they are doing wrong, and that is funding congresses and other things" (Mauro).
> "They have a budget for that. They have to select who they're going to give it to." (Mauro).
> "Because what do they do? They open up the prospect to the doctor. They go up to 'so-and-so' and say: Look, if you prescribe such-and-such a drug 'legally', we're going to send you to Congress X. And the guy starts prescribing the drug. They start like that" (Mauro).
> "Sometimes it's even the doctor who asks. You say to the guy, for example: Well, can't you get a Congress for me, in Florianopolis or wherever? Well, you're not prescribing the medicine properly... Al, the guy prescribes the medicine... Sometimes it has indications, and if he prescribes it with indications, it's 'less bad'" (Mauro).

Negotiating prescriptions in exchange for funding for congresses or any other benefits has become commonplace in the interaction between doctors and the pharmaceutical industry. With the focus of the problem redirected towards whether or not to prescribe, there has also been a relativization of the important ethical aspects involved in this practice.

> "[...] A large proportion of doctors [...] start prescribing the product to please [...], to be harassed by the representative" (Mauro).
> "[...] what we see in practice is this: Many doctors prescribe medication unnecessarily" (Mauro).
> "[...] the majority [of doctors] really go with the flow, delude themselves, prescribe a drug inappropriately" (Mauro).
> "I know a cardiologist who went to Turkey for a European congress because he was the one who prescribed the drug the most" (Mauro).
> "For the representative, it's good because it increases sales in the region. The guy is using the drug, it's great for him" (Mauro).
> "So we criticize that. Not medication without an indication. I think you have to take the medication at the right time" (Mauro).
> "I prescribe because it's valid, it's good for the patient, but it's never controlled by the representative" (Mauro).
> "[...] a study has come out with a substance saying that it prevents diabetes. But you're not allowed to take it for patients who aren't diabetic yet. Then you see a lot of guys doing it to prevent diabetes. And he's fine with the lab" (Mauro).

Still on the subject of funding for participation in congresses, the doctor interviewed reports a competition between the various pharmaceutical industries, the background to which is prescription. It also helps to understand the industry's strategic interest in the university environment. To the extent that the reputation of academia is a benchmark for quality, this partnership fosters prescriptive credibility.

> "[...] They, from [the laboratory] Norvartis, sent a drug [...] and said: [...] if you prescribe this drug for 80 patients, you will go to San Francisco for the Congress [...]" (Mauro).
> "So I'm never going to that Congress, because I'm not going to prescribe this for 80 patients. I won't be able to do that... (laughing)" (Mauro).
> "Then the people from Merck [...] said: Oh, the people from Sao Paulo have sent to invite you to the Congress in San Francisco" (Mauro).
> "Then the guy [from Norvartis] arrived, and I said: Now I'm not going to prescribe for 80, because Merck invited me" (Mauro).
> "Really? Then let's see what I can do for you..." (Mauro).
> "They come with a lot behind them because, in practice, we [...] influence prescribing a lot. Sometimes you don't prescribe much, but the guy sees you prescribing, and he starts prescribing too" (Mauro).
> "Sometimes I go to a laboratory congress. We go to a lot of these conferences. But here at the University, it's because you replicate; it's different" (Mauro).
> "The guy doesn't focus on whether you're prescribing it. And because, as they say: you're a replicator of information, and that's interesting to them, in a way" (Mauro).

In refresher and continuing education programs, the strategy for disseminating medicines is based on lectures given by opinion leaders, located by their leadership role in their respective regions. With a profile well defined by the pharmaceutical industry, the speaker transmits research results on medicines. A paid contract is established and, before each talk, the speaker takes part in a meeting with industry promoters to prepare in advance what he is going to present.

> "[...] The trend is very much to keep up to date. [...] they do a survey in the area and take people from the region. That's basically the opinion leader" (Mauro).
> "At these meetings, the doctor starts to see where he can use that medicine" (Mauro).
> "And they look for lecturers from the university a lot" (Mauro).
> "[...] they select a lot. And a person who is зёпа, who works with research, who can transmit information well, who transmits seriousness and who transmits something they know" (Mauro)
> "The industry invites you and they [the laboratory staff] hold a meeting. Then we prepare to present some things" (Mauro).
> "If he goes there to talk about a certain medicine, [...] the laboratory, in theory, will pay for at least part of his stay" (Luis).
> "It's all paid, really paid. It's all down to them: plane tickets, hotels, they pick you up and take you away" (Mauro).
> "There are companies [...] that work together with the laboratory, just to bring in lecturers" (Mauro).

It is in the speeches explaining the content of the lectures that the conflict of interests becomes most evident. Here we can see a polemic that goes beyond the interests of health care, as well as the priority of the therapeutic perspective, to fall into a logic of commercial commitment to the agency funding the event. Without the freedom to reliably disclose the data on the drug presented, such as side effects and contraindications, the speaker calls into question the credibility of knowledge. And, with great effort, he tries to make his speech impartial, making it clear that he is not there to advertise for the pharmaceutical industry.

> "At the congresses I've been to, [...] the presenter, before presenting any lecture, any data, any medicine, presents a slide that says whether it was funded by a laboratory, which laboratories, which interests are linked or not to that presentation" (Luis).

"There is no [...] construction of a critical matrix on the introduction of new drugs, [...] from a non 'commercial' point of view, access to the new knowledge generated in this research" (Tc3ë).
"And when you take part in a study like this, they end up getting you to talk about the study" (Mauro)
"Even if he doesn't talk about the commercial name, he's going to talk about a drug that, in theory, he's going to try to bring up the benefits of the drug. But that doesn't exempt them from talking about the side effects" (Luis).
"If I'm going to talk about these studies, I'm going to say that the other [statin] also reduces it, which is independent of the drug. I'm not going to advertise the guy who's funding me to present that product. I'm going to say that the other one does it too, right?" (Mauro).

Although there is reference to the critical aspect of the presentation, when the speakers refer to criticism, they are referring to the possibility of opposing, or not, the pressures of the pharmaceutical industry. This means a shift away from concern about the legitimate efficacy of the product, supposedly proven in clinical trials. It implies a position in defense of the drug that involves ethically questionable values; an approach that even relativizes the possibility of omitting data related to side effects and contraindications of the drug presented.

"Nowadays, we joke that Statistics is the art of torturing numbers so that they confess what we want. You put it the way you want it" (Mauro).
"So we have to be very critical. When I give a talk, I'm very honest. [...] I'm not going to say something that I don't think is true" (Mauro).
"For example, I attended a lecture where the guy's graph didn't have the 0 point, making it clear that it was a way of manipulating information in statistical terms" (S'rgio).
"Look, they [the lab staff] never put me off anything. [...] they even like you to put it on... because then it sounds real" (Mauro).
"Today, conflict of interest is an issue that everyone considers. If someone is going to present a paper that has been funded by the laboratory, that's the first thing they talk about. They talk about the benefits of the drug, but they also talk about the side effects and contraindications" (Crgio).
"I went to give a talk about rimonabant (Acomplia®) and I said that there's a risk of depression, there's a risk of suicidal ideas." (Mauro).
"[...] But if you say: Ah, rimonabant makes you want to kill yourself. Or] the statin can cause liver damage... [it gets complicated]" (Mauro). [it gets complicated]" (Mauro).

Under the guidance of pharmaceutical industry coordinators, some arguments recur in doctors' speeches and are part of a rehearsed discourse. Their aim is to minimize the existence of side effects and product contraindications.

> "For some time now, [...] clinical research has been more concerned with patient safety. [...] with the demonstration of adverse effects in large populations, clinical trials have taken a closer look at drug toxicity" (Josd).
> "A patient of mine [...] had been taking a statin. [...] she had drug hepatitis and the doctor said it was the statin." (Mauro).
> "[...] I was taking Norfloxacin [...]; the biggest risk is hepatitis. It's very high, but everyone prescribes it" (Mauro).
> "[...] It's much easier to say it was the statin; not the quinolone [...] to treat the urinary infection. [...] How many percent of people who take statins suffer liver damage? - 1%. The other is more than 50" (Mauro).

In order to dismantle difficulties in sales potential, there is a ready-made package of information to be presented by the speakers, whose strategy is based on comparing products being launched with drugs already consolidated on the market. With the intention of similarly demolishing restrictions on their use, such as statins, they cite substances such as aspirin, anesthetics, penicillin and other antibiotics, in order to say that, despite their potentially known side effects, the prescribing practice of these drugs remains unchallenged.

> "I usually show a slide that we have there: Look at aspirin, everyone takes it, and it has a risk of causing bleeding. In every 200 (two hundred) patients, 1 (one) can have a hemorrhage. In less than 1000 (one thousand) patients, 1 (one) can have a fatal hemorrhage. [But] everyone prescribes aspirin" (Mauro).
> "And of course we can have side effects, but that's part of the show" (Luis).
> "Of course, you use penicillin. How many patients die from using penicillin? Have you stopped using penicillin?" (Luis).
> "How many anaphylactic shocks are there because of anesthetics? Do you stop operating on patients because of that? That's part of the game" (Luis).
> "Whereas for a statin to cause liver damage or something else, it's over a million times more. So we analyze and see that you could really be taking a drug that everyone thinks is a trivial matter, but which could be causing a risk" (Mauro).

The dissemination and promotion of medicines through representatives of the pharmaceutical industry appear to be the main alternative to the difficulty of "cutting edge" doctors (outside academic centers) to keep up to date with medical-scientific progress.

> "*It*'s difficult for the doctor who's working in the clinic to subscribe to a magazine to keep up to date. So it's the representatives who really bring the knowledge to him" (Mauro).
> "They arrive with articles, sometimes a booklet; they ask if the doctor wants one article or another" (Mauro).

A number of aspects have been raised regarding interference in medical prescribing, including the role of sales reps as strategic promoters of medicines. Through direct contact with doctors, they act as spokespeople for the interests of pharmaceutical companies, directing information to influence prescribing habits. In the name of science, they present studies on the indications of drugs whose use has not yet been approved in Brazil.

> "The laboratory, through its representatives, can even try to interfere with the prescription" (Sergio).
> "And the representative is not a doctor, he is charged directly by his manager. He has to sell" (Mauro).
> "In fact, they don't put out an indication, they present a study; they give lectures presenting the study. But it hasn't been approved for use yet" (Mauro).
> "For example, there is a medicine that has already been released in the United States [...] and is in use there. [...] Until recently, people were importing it to use. [...] the medicine is now being used without having been approved here" (Mauro).

Another aspect of this discussion concerns the manipulation of the indication of the substance. In this sense, the representatives are trained to strategically present the drugs, pointing out therapeutic possibilities that extend to other specialties, "playing into the hands" of the professionals, in order to increase their sales potential.

> "[...] In practice, the representative arrives with that news for the top doctor; he doesn't get carried away, but that information is passed on in meetings" (Mauro.)
> "[...] The intention of the laboratory is often not for the doctor to use the

> medicine unnecessarily" (Mauro).
> "[...] a drug [...] that increases insulin sensitivity. They fell for the cardiologists, and [they] started treating diabetes, massively prescribing the drug. And that increases the sales power" (Mauro).
> "I say: stop encouraging the cardiologist [...], they won't know how to use the medicine, and that ends up destroying the medicine" (Mauro).
> "The laboratory gains a lot from this, because it's prescription without indication. So they earn a lot" (Mauro).
> "The conflict of interest needs to be identified by the doctor who is disclosing a result. They are potential conflicts" (Тсзё).

Despite the sharpness of these speeches, it is possible to perceive, in the intertext of their content, a minimization of the biased conduct of the pharmaceutical industries. Through a strange counterpoint, "the doctor's head" is placed in the place of responsibility for what happens. This points to a relativization of such magnitude in prescriptive practice that it destabilizes medicine as a defensible pillar of ethical-political-social values.

> "There are different views: [...] it may be encouraging consumption, but it also [...] creates greater responsibility for health professionals, whether they are prescribing correctly or not" (Тсвё).
> "[...] some laboratories are aware of this and don't want us to say that it's okay to use it, as if it were water with sugar. It's not like that. There are indications!" (Mauro).
> "The important thing is that you work this into the doctor's head. That the medicine has to be used at the right time, in the right way" (Mauro).
> "[...] the doctor has to have the good sense to know how to discern this; when to prescribe and when not to prescribe, which is something that has to be defined" (Mauro).
> "Sometimes there's another problem, which is the cost. Sometimes his [the representative's] medicine is more expensive. And there's another one that's cheaper and works just as well. So the guy stops prescribing that one, you know?" (Mauro).
> "So there is [...] interest from the doctor, and also interest from the laboratory, which is joining in. [...] They [the representatives] are beginning to be aware of this. In practice, this ends up burning" (Mauro).
> "Doctors have to know that it's not a drug to prescribe to just anyone. Now, there are doctors who are already using it indiscriminately" (Mauro).

As discussed in the chapter on power, Foucault's concept of the inseparability of the knowledge/power relationship is clearly relevant. In this sense, it is worth noting the alliance between the economic power of the pharmaceutical industry and legal knowledge in the contemporary configuration of power. Given the indisputable ethical parameters involved in the production and dissemination of medical knowledge, it is essential to note, based on the testimony below, the potential triggering of compensation mechanisms as part of a process of judicialization of politics. Functioning as a prescriptive control mechanism, this means that the political dimension has been replaced by individual legal appeals.

> "[...] many times, a remedy that is effective for a certain category of patients, with a certain disease, would not have that care if that knowledge did not reach the population" (Jose).
> "[...] we are living in an era in which the consumer himself is becoming more active" (Jose).
> "There is [...] a window of opportunity [...], the claims for compensation: either because the doctor failed to prescribe what he should have prescribed on the basis of scientific evidence, or because the doctor prescribed something that there was no need to prescribe, or because the health system is not providing what it should to the patient" (Jose).

Linked to the economic interests of the pharmaceutical industry, there is a dynamic in which patient, consumer and citizen, representatively amalgamated, have come to actively participate in the process of collectivizing scientific knowledge. If, on the one hand, this increases the autonomy of discussion, on the other, it makes consumers' heads spin. If the prescription doesn't correspond to what they expect, the patient looks for another doctor.

In the contemporary configuration of power, this process corresponds to the end of the disciplinary society and the installation of the control society. Discipline, which used to be directed at bodies, now encompasses the very identity of subjects - permanently reconstructed by the media and technological updates.

This is the biopolitical dimension of power which, when exercised, limits the supposed social omnipotence of medicine and colonizes the medical profession. In the context of the influence of the pharmaceutical industry's economic power, this reinforces the perspective through which the doctor is stripped of exclusive decision-making power.

By assimilating the relationship between the pharmaceutical industry and the prescribing doctor as an inseparable binomial, the discourse below gives expression to a non-dogmatic view of the issue, discouraging the inhibition or liberalization of either party to the "conflict" and believing in the possibility of transparency in this interaction.

> "There will always be a conflict of interest in the binomial. The pharmaceutical industry wants to make a profit from the drug being researched, and the doctor who took part is thrilled with the results, which have meant that treatment has progressed" (Jose).
> "The conflict of interest exists in various forms. The direct form: the industry pressures the consumer network to use by publishing in the lay media [...]. The indirect form: by promoting dissemination" (Josd).
> "[...] we have to look at this in a non-dogmatic way. Only now are we beginning to understand the details of this relationship. And what inhibiting on the one hand and liberalizing in a profound way on the other could do to any system" (Josd).
> "[...] it's important [...] to look at it as more than just right and wrong, [...] and turn it into something transparent" (Jose).
> "What is fundamental is that academia, medical societies, doctors, teachers and all health professionals can understand that there is nothing in this relationship that cannot be discussed" (Jose).

As you can see, the way in which the problem is perceived tends to minimize the indisputable and important ethical aspects involved in the process.

## Final considerations

This paper is the result of an investigation carried out at a public university hospital into the links between the pharmaceutical industry and the knowledge industry. The investigation generated conclusions that suggest that the scientific legitimization of pharmaceutical industry products is based on attracting collaborating doctors who are willing to join research projects. It is worth pointing out that a possible limitation of this study is the relative limitation of the number of interviews, restricted to professionals from the same institution, which suggests caution regarding the possible extrapolation of empirical findings to broader contexts. Even so, I would emphasize the consistency of what was observed with what is reported in the literature, as well as with what the medical field itself, of which I am a part, points out.

The analysis and discussion of the testimonies showed that, in the sample studied, the co-construction of medical knowledge with medical professors is a powerful marketing strategy for the pharmaceutical industry. This means that the industry strategically relies on the results of this interaction to expand the consumption of its medicines. To the extent that the interest in disseminating knowledge is related to the prescribing potential of the drug, the industry assigns the role of prescribing technician to the doctor, making him the main target of its marketing strategies.

The analysis of empirical data related to the role of the industry in financing the production of medical knowledge was based on the way in which doctors are involved in research and the process of building clinical evidence. The results showed that, in the contracts established with the industry, collaborating doctors are paid per patient recruited or by a previously stipulated monthly amount. The clinical trial protocols for testing new drugs are drawn up by the sponsoring industry without the participation of the collaborating doctor. The data collected is sent in its raw state to be analyzed by the sponsor, i.e. access to the full data collected is exclusive to the central coordinators of the research. And the results of the trials, presented in abstracts, are previously subjected to data selection criteria.

Corroborated by Guimaraes (2007), these data mean that, in most processes of co-production of clinical evidence, the participation of doctors in research does not go beyond the inclusion of patients and the execution of procedures provided for in a standardized protocol. In this context of manipulation, the publication of articles containing research results is also under the absolute power of pharmaceutical industry interests.

As mentioned in the previous chapter, the merit of scientific contributions, considered from a category called "impact", is indicated by the number of times the article is cited in indexed journals. According to Guimaraes (2007), "of the 25 publications in the human health sector with more than 250 citations, 13 are multicenter clinical trials testing new drugs or procedures" (p.19), and are therefore considered to have a high "impact". This means that the "impact" is strongly influenced by the way in which the research was organized: with large networks of researchers with the potential to attract patients who submit to standardized protocols; with researchers being paid per patient attracted; and without guaranteeing the ethical standards of research (GUIMARAES, 2007).

It is worth remembering that, when discussing the power of the pharmaceutical industry in the production of medical knowledge, Angell (2007) highlights the industry's influence on medical research by saying that "the clear aim was to bias the data to ensure that their drugs performed well" (p.16). With obvious manipulation of the original research writers, the pharmaceutical industry hires *ghost-writers* to sign off on studies in which they did not participate.

These "results", as well as being published, are disseminated to prescribing doctors - at congresses, specialization courses or continuing education - by speakers trained by the pharmaceutical industry's marketing coordinators. In this way, the content and presentation of new drugs, as well as their clinical indications, have become strategies for interfering in doctors' prescribing practices.

Biologically based, the style of medical thinking is used strategically by opinion formers to bias results and interfere in doctors' prescriptive practices. In the midst of the forces of economic power, this contradiction is magnified to the exact extent that the processes of medical knowledge production, dominated by biology and epidemiology, are beyond the critical capacity of most doctors.

In view of the conflicts of interest involved in the production of medical knowledge, it is worth highlighting the vulnerability of doctors who, due to deficiencies in their own training, are not trained to critically evaluate the research results presented by the pharmaceutical industry. It is enough for the study to be attributed scientific legitimacy for the doctor to blindly believe the information it contains. This susceptibility of doctors to assimilating any information from the scientific world as true should be considered worrying, because in this way doctors are subjected to a process of passive assimilation of knowledge.

In this context of dominant power techniques, between collaborating doctors and the pharmaceutical industry, the co-production of medical knowledge is outlined as a relationship of domination. Subjected to strategic power techniques, the role of the doctor has become that of a power technician. Because they are strategic and powerful, these mechanisms take advantage of points of medical vulnerability. This points to a relativization of such magnitude in prescriptive practice that it destabilizes medicine as a defensible pillar of ethical-political-social values.

On the other hand, considering that the doctor's interaction with the pharmaceutical industry is based on the possibility of co-constructing research projects, it is precisely the perspective of this co-construction that gives consistency to, and makes possible, an approach to the doctor's ethical commitment. This means that the mere participation of the doctor in a "pharmaceutical industry project" implies that the doctor is involved in the ethical issue, since the role of power technician does not relieve him of the responsibility of legitimate knowledge.

Whether as an explicit message or as an intertextual figure of speech, this is the aspect that intertwines ethical, political and scientific forces in the epistemological field of medicine. However, despite these conflicts of interest, the analysis of the testimonies showed that, in this sphere of apprehension, doctors' conceptions exclude the indisputable ethical aspects involved in the process. An example of this is the explanatory discourse on the content of the lectures, which goes beyond the interests of care and the therapeutic perspective, to fall into a logic of commercial commitment to the funding agency. By minimizing the biased conduct of the pharmaceutical industry, the speaker calls into question the credibility of the knowledge presented.

It is therefore a composition of power that limits the supposed social omnipotence of medicine, while at the same time colonizing the medical profession. In this sense, the critical and reflective capacity of the prescribing doctor gains in importance, both in terms of their professional practices and their ability to assess the quality of the medical knowledge presented as new. On the other hand, as far as the pharmaceutical industry is concerned, Guimaraes (2007) argues that the funding of clinical trials should not be discouraged or restrained, "as long as ethical standards and republican practices of remuneration per patient captured are guaranteed".

It is important to emphasize that, without demonizing social roles, it is possible to read the forgas field based on the quality and ambiguity of these forgas, and not just by measuring their intensity. It is with this critical eye that this study can conclude. With the aim of linking medical knowledge to market expectations, the dominant power is exercised through power techniques (marketing strategies), giving doctors the role of power technicians at the service of their interests. In the contemporary configuration of power, there is therefore a relativization of values that calls for a critical ethical review.

## References

ABRAMSON, John. **Overdosed America**: the broken promise of American medicine. New York: H. Perenium, 2005. 167p.

ADAM, Philippe, HERZLICH, Claudine. **Sociology of illness and medicine**. Sao Paulo: EDUSC, 2001. 144p.

ANDREAZZI, M. F.; KORNIS, G. Transformations and challenges of private health care in Brazil in the 90s. **Physis**, Rio de Janeiro, v. 13, n. 1, p. 157-191, 2003.

ANGELL, Marcia. **The truth about pharmaceutical laboratories**: how we are deceived and what we can do about it. Rio de Janeiro: Record, 2007. 319p.

ARAGAO, E.; BARROS, E.; OLIVEIRA, S. Talando de metodologia de pesquisa. **Estudos e Pesquisas em Psicologia**, Rio de Janeiro, Year 5, n. 2, 2005.

ATIVUS to expand production. **Gazeta Mercantil,** Sao Paulo, December 12, 2007. This was reported in the press. Available at: <http//www.gazetamercantil.com.br>. Accessed on: Feb. 25, 2008.

BECKER, Howard. **Research Methods in the Social Sciences**. Sao Paulo: Hucitec, 1993. 178p.

BERNAL, J. D. International Science. In: BERNAL. J. D. **The social function of science**. Cambridge, Massachusetts: MIT, 1964. p. 200-237.

BIRMAN, Joel. Archives of biopolitics. In: LOYOLA, M. A. **Bioethics:** reproduction and gender in contemporary society. ABEP/LETRAS LIVRES, 2005, p. 27-48.

BLANK, Nelson. **Clinical reasoning and medical equipment**: subsidies for understanding the significance of diagnostic and therapeutic equipment for medicine. 1985. Dissertation (Master's in Collective Health)-Institute of Social Medicine, Rio de Janeiro State University, Rio de Janeiro, 1985.

BOBBIO, Norberto. **State, government, society**: towards a general theory of politics. Sao Paulo: Paz e Terra, 2004. 173p.

BONET, Octavio. **Knowing and feeling**: an ethnography of learning biomedicine. 1996. Dissertation (Master's Degree in Social Anthropology)-National Museum, Federal University of Rio de Janeiro, Rio de Janeiro, 1996.

BOURDIEU, Pierre. The scientific field. In: ORTIZ, R. (Org.) **Bourdieu**. Sao Paulo: Atica, 1973.

. **O poder simbolico**. Rio de Janeiro: Bertrand Brasil, 2005. 311p.

BRAZIL. Ministry of Health. **Information Portal of the National STD and AIDS Program**. Available at: <http//www.aids.gov.br>. Accessed on: 03 Nov. 2007.

BRAUDEL, Fernand. **The dynamics of capitalism**. Rio de Janeiro: Rocco, 1987. 94p.

CAMARGO JUNIOR, Kenneth. **Biomedicine, knowledge & science**: a critical approach. Sao Paulo: Hucitec, 2003. 195p.

. Epistemology at a time like this?: the limits of care. In: PINHEIRO, R.; MATTOS, R. (Org.). **Cuidado**: as fronteiras da integralidade. Rio de Janeiro: Hucitec/ABRASCO, 2004. p. 157-170.

**Medical (Ir)rationality**: the paradoxes of the clinic. 1990. Dissertation (Masters in Collective Health)-Institute of Social Medicine, Rio de Janeiro State University, Rio de Janeiro, 1990.

. **Medicine, medicalization and symbolic production**. In: PITTA, A. (Org.) **Saude & Comunicação:** visibilidades e silencios, Sao Paulo/Rio de Janeiro, Hucitec/ABRASCO, 1995, p. 13-24.

. **The political economy of the production and diffusion of biomedical knowledge**, 2007. Mimeo.

CAMPOS, F.; AGUIAR, R. Basic care and curricular reform. In: NEGRI, B.; FARIA, Rua; VIANA, A. (Org.). **Recursos humanos em saude**: política, desenvolvimento e mercado de trabalho. Sao Paulo: Unicamp, 2002. p. 91-99.

CANGUILHEM, George. **The normal and the pathological**. 6. ed. Rio de Janeiro: Forense Universitaria, 2006. 293p.

CLAVREUL, Jean. **The medical order**: the power and powerlessness of medical discourse. Sao Paulo: Brasiliense, 1978. 273p.

CONSUMERS INTERNATIONAL. **Drugs, doctors and dinners**: how drug companies influence health in the developing world. Oct. 2007. Available at: <http//www.consumersinternational.org>. Accessed on: Nov. 10, 2007.

CORDEIRO, Hesio. **Determinants of drug consumption**. 1978. Dissertation (Master's Degree in Social Medicine)-Institute of Social Medicine, Rio de Janeiro State University, Rio de Janeiro, 1978.

DAIN, S.; SOARES, L. State reform and public policies: intergovernmental relations and decentralization since 1988. In: AZEREDO, B; OLIVEIRA, M. A. de (Org.). **State reform and employment policies in Brazil**. Campinas:

Unicamp/Institute of Economics, 1998.

DELEUZE, Gilles. **Foucault**. Sao Paulo: Brasiliense, 1988. 142p.

DOBB, M. **The evolution of capitalism**. Rio de Janeiro: LTC, 1987. 396p.

FAVORETO, C.; CAMARGO JUNIOR, K. Some conceptual and technical-operational challenges for the development of the Family Health Program as a proposal to transform the care model. **Physis**, Rio de Janeiro, v. 12, n.1, p. 62-71, 2002.

FISHER, W. **Science-USA**: the politics of ignorance. New York: Envolverde/IPS, 2006.

FLECK, L. **Genesis and development of a scientific fact**. Chicago: University of Chicago, 1979. 203 p.

FOUCAULT, Michel. **The archaeology of knowledge**. 7. ed. Rio de Janeiro: Forense Universitaria, 2007. 236p.

. Lecture January 7, 1976. In: FOUCAULT, Michel. **In defense of society**. Sao Paulo: Martins Fontes, 2002. p. 3-26.

. **Microphysics of power**. Rio de Janeiro: Graal, 1995. 295p.

. **The birth of the clinic**. 5. ed. Rio de Janeiro: Forense Universitaria, 1998. 241p.

. The birth of social medicine. In: FOUCAULT, Michel. **The microphysics of power**. Rio de Janeiro: Graal, 1995. Chap. V, p. 79-98.

. The birth of the hospital. In: FOUCAULT, Michel. **The microphysics of power**. Rio de Janeiro: Graal, 1995. Chap. VI, p. 99-111.

. **Words and things**. 4. ed. São Paulo: Martins Fontes, 1987. 405p.

. **Summary of courses at the College de France (1970-1982).** Rio de Janeiro: J. Zahar, 1997. 134p.

GADELHA, C. The health industrial complex and the need for a dynamic approach to health economics. **Ciencia & Saude Coletiva**, Rio de Janeiro, v. 8, n. 2, p. 521-35, 2003.

GINZBURG, Carlo. Signs: the roots of an indicative paradigm. In: GINZBURG, C. **Myths, emblems, signs:** morphology and history. São Paulo: Companhia das Letras, 1989, p. 143-179.

GOLDIM, J. R. Conflicts of interest and their repercussions on science. **Revista Brasileira de Psiquiatria**, Sao Paulo, v. 28, n. 1, 2006. Available at: <http://www.ufrgs.br/bioetica/conflit.htm>. Accessed on: December 12, 2007.

GOOD, Byron. How medicine constructs its objects. In: GOOD, B. **Medicine, rationality and experience an anthropological perspective**. Cambridge, UK: Cambridge University Press, 1999. Chap.3, p. 65-197.

GREENE, Jeremy. **Prescribing by numbers**: drugs and definition of disease. Maryland, USA: Johns Hopkins University Press, 2007. 309p.

GUATTARI, Felix. **Chaosmosis**: a new aesthetic paradigm. Rio de Janeiro: Vozes, 1992. 203p.

. **Molecular revolution**: political pulsations of desire. 3. ed. Sao Paulo: Brasiliense, 1987. 226p.

GUATTARI, F.; ROLNIK, S. **Micropolftica**: cartographies of desire. 7. ed. rev. Petropolis: Vozes, 2005. 436p.

GUEDES, C.; NOGUEIRA, M. I.; CAMARGO JUNIOR, K. Subjectivity as anomaly: epistemological contributions to the critique of the biomedical model. **Ciencia & Saude Coletiva**, Rio de Janeiro, v. 11, n. 4, p. 1093-1103, 2006.

GUERREIRO, Iara. **Report of the meeting on ethics in qualitative health research**. Sao Paulo: Municipal Health Department, Ethics Committee, 2007.

GUIMARAES, R. Quality, impact and citation: an obscure relationship. **Radis**, Rio de Janeiro, n.55, 2007. Available at : <http://www.ensp.fiocruz.br/radis/55/postudo.html>. Accessed on: September 18, 2007.

HABERMAS, Jurgen. **Technology and science as "ideology"**. Lisbon: Edigoes 70, 1968. 147p.

HACKING, I.: **The emergency of probability**: a philosophical study of early ideas about probability, induction and statistical inference. UK: Cambridge University Press, 1975. Chap. 4, p. 31-48.

. Language, truth and reason. In: HOLLIS, M., STEVEN, L. (Org.). **Rationality and relativism**. Cambridge, Mass.: MIT Press, 1982. p. 49-66.

. **The social construction of what?** Cambridge, Mass.: Harvard University Press, 2000. 124p.

HARDT, M.; NEGRI, A. **Imperio**. Rio de Janeiro: Record, 2001. 501p.

HEALY, D. The latest mania: selling bipolar disorder. **PloS Medicine**, v. 3, n. 4, 2006.

HESS, David. The cultural construction of science and technology. In: HESS, D.

**Science and technology in a multicultural world**. New York: Columbia Univ. Press, 1995. p. 52-53.

HOBBES, Thomas. **Leviathan**. Sao Paulo: Martin Claret, 2004. 519p.

HOCHMAN, Gilberto. Science between the community and the market: readings of Kuhn, Bourdieu, Latour and Knorr-Cetina. In: PORTOCARRERO, V. (Org.). **Filosofia, historia e sociologia das ciencias**. Rio de Janeiro: Fiocruz, 2002. Chap. 8, p. 199-230.

KNORR-CETINA, Karen. The scientist as a socially situated reasoner: from scientific communities to transcientific fields. In: KNORR-CETINA, K. **The manufacture of knowledge**: an essay on the constructivists and contextual nature of science. Oxford: Pergamon, 1981. p. 68-93.

LEXCHIN, Joel. Bigger and better: how Pfizer redefined erectile dysfunction. **PloS Medicine**, 2006, v. 3, n. 4. Available at: <www.plosmedicine.org>. Accessed on: January 29, 2007.

MAGGINI, M.; VANACORE, N.; RASCHETTI, R. Cholinesterase inhibitors: drugs looking for a disease? **PloS Medicine**, v. 3, n. 4. p.140, 2006.

MATTOS, Ruben. The meanings of comprehensiveness: some reflections on values that deserve to be defended. In: PINHEIRO, R., MATTOS, R. (Org.). **Os sentidos da integralidade**: na atencao e no cuidado a saude. Rio de Janeiro: UERJ, IMS: ABRASCO, 2001. p. 39-64.

MINAYO, Maria Cecilia. **The challenge of knowledge**: qualitative research in health. Sao Paulo: Hucitec, 1992. 269p.

MOYNIHAN, R. The making of a disease: female sexual dysfunction. **British**

**Medical Journal**, Washington, v. 326, 2003. Available at: <http//www.bmj.com>. Accessed on: January 29, 2007.

MOYNIHAN, R.; HENRY, D. The fight against disease mongering: generating knowledge for action. **PloS Medicine,** 2006, v. 3, n. 4, e191.

MULKAY, Michael. **Science and the wider society**. In: MULKAY, M. **Science and the sociology of knowledge**. London: Allen & Unwin, 1979. p. 97-129.

PAYER, Lynn. The major disease-mongering tactics identified by Lynn Payer. Box 1. In: TIEFER, L. **Female sexual dysfunction**: a case study of disease mongering and activist resistance. **PloS Medicine**, 2006, v. 3, n. 4, e178.

PELBART, Peter Pal. **Capital life**. Sao Paulo: Iluminuras, 2003. p. 252.

PHILLIPS, Christine. Medicine goes to school: teachers as sickness brokers for ADHD. **PloS Medicine**, 2006, v. 3, n. 4, e182.

POLANYI, Karl. **The great transformation**: the origins of our epoch. Rio de Janeiro: Elsevier, 2000. 349p.

SANTOS, Boaventura de Sousa. **A discourse on the sciences**. 3. ed. Sao Paulo: Cortez, 2005. 92p.

SAYD, Jane. **Mediar, medicar, remediar**: aspectos da terapeutica na medicina ocidental. Rio de Janeiro: EdUERJ, 1998. 193p.

. **Origins of contemporary medicine**: a brief review. Rio de Janeiro: UFRJ, 1998 (Series Studies in Collective Health, n. 173).

. **Being a doctor**: a historical perspective. Rio de Janeiro: UERJ/IMS, 2006 (Series

Studies in Collective Health, n. 220).

SEGATTO, Cristiane. The toast is not free. **Revista Epoca**, Rio de Janeiro, issue no. 495, p. 114, Nov. 2007. Segao Health and Wellness Ethics.

SPINK, M. J. Researching in everyday life: recovering memories of research in social psychology. **Psicologia & Sociedade**, Sao Paulo, v. 19, n. 1, p. 7-14, 2007.

SPINK, M. J.; MEDRADO, B.; PASSARELLI, C. A. et al. **Praticas discursivas e produgao de sentidos no cotidiano**: aproximagoes teoricas e metodologicas. 3. ed. Sao Paulo: Cortez, 2004. 293p.

STEINMAN, M.; BERO, L.; CHREN, M-M.; LANDERFELD, C. Narrative review: the promotion of Gabapentin: an analysis of internal industry documents. **Annals of Internal Medicine**, v. 145, n. 4, 2006, p. 284-293.

TIEFER, Leonore. Female sexual dysfunction: a case study of disease mongering and activist resistance. **PloS Medicine**, 2006, v. 3, n. 4. Available at: <www.plosmedicine.org>. Accessed on: Jan. 29, 2007.

VIANNA, Cid Manso de Mello. Structures of the health system: from the medical-industrial complex to the medical-financial complex. **Physis**, Rio de Janeiro, v. 12, n. 2,л 375390, 2002.

WEISZ, George. From clinical counting to evidence-based medicine In: Jorland, G.; Opinel, A. (Org.). **Body counts**: medical quantification in historical and sociological perspectives. London: McGill-Queens Press, 2005.

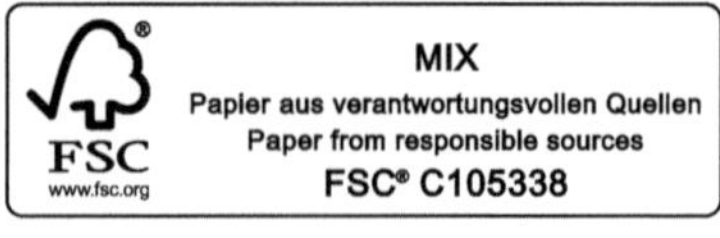


Printed by Books on Demand GmbH, Norderstedt / Germany